Children with Gender Identity Disorder

Routledge Studies in Health and Social Welfare

Children with Gender Identity Disorder

A Clinical, Ethical, and Legal Analysis

Simona Giordano

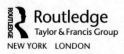
Routledge
Taylor & Francis Group
NEW YORK   LONDON

First published 2013
by Routledge
711 Third Avenue, New York, NY 10017

Simultaneously published in the UK
by Routledge
2 Park Square, Milton Park, Abingdon, Oxon OX14 4RN

*Routledge is an imprint of the Taylor & Francis Group,
an informa business*

Library of Congress Cataloging-in-Publication Data
Giordano, Simona, Dr.
   Children with gender identity disorder : a clinical, ethical, and legal
analysis / by Simona Giordano.
      p. cm. — (Routledge studies in health and social welfare)
   Includes bibliographical references and index.
   1. Gender identity disorders in children—Social aspects.   2. Gender
identity disorders in children—Counseling of.   3. Gender identity
disorders in children—Moral and ethical aspects.   I. Title.
   RJ506.G35G67 2012
   618.928583—dc23
   2012008698

ISBN13: 978-0-415-50271-9 (hbk)
ISBN13: 978-0-203-09789-2 (ebk)

Typeset in Sabon
by IBT Global.

Printed and bound in the United States of America on sustainably sourced
paper by IBT Global.

To the disobedient servants

Contents

Foreword

John Harris

Simona Giordano has written a beautiful and complex book, a compassionate, humane, elegant, and poetic book, about vulnerable and often violated people. This is a book few could or would have written, but of which anyone would be proud.

Dr. Giordano is a philosopher by training and a poet in spirit, and in writing about the predicament, condition, feelings, and lives of transgender individuals she deploys not only considerable philosophical and analytical skills, but does justice to other literatures: psychological, sociological, legal, medical, and artistic. The book draws on sources in all these fields as illustrative of her text and as grist to the argument, enriching our understanding and sharpening our insight.

I cannot think of a book quite like this. It defies classification, and yet by the power of its argument, the imagination of its conception, and the wealth of apposite examples and illustrations, it compels attention and surely shapes our understanding for the better. And by this I mean to include better morally and better in the sense of compelling a more rounded and sympathetic appreciation of both the complexity of the issues and the depth of understanding of the human dimension of that too often seen as a medical issue or indeed simply an issue of misguided preference.

Giordano's book begins with a quotation from Fabrizio de André's "And like all the most beautiful things, you lived one day only, like a rose". André gives his heroine twenty-three hours more than Shakespeare with a related thought:

> "For women are as roses, whose fair flower
> Being once display'd, doth fall that very hour".[1]

But André's image is purer and more unequivocally sympathetic; Shakespeare's has somewhat coarse and deliberate sexual allusions, for all its sonorous beauty of expression. What Giordano has achieved is the capture and celebration of the beauty of people in sad and wretched circumstances, and the nobility, not of suffering (there is nothing noble about that, ignoble rather), but the nobility of the minorities, who are often forced into unnecessary suffering for no other reason than their powerlessness. It is this exploration of the nobility of transgender youth, who are often vulnerable and disadvantaged, and of the ways in which the painful necessity of exhibiting that nobility can be removed or mitigated which is the great strength and the overwhelming virtue of this book.

I will not here rehearse the books' subject matter; that is well set out in the Table of Contents which precedes this foreword.

Simona Giordano is a genuinely brilliant and original philosopher whose highly distinctive and important work on eating disorders, exercise, and gender is simply the best of its kind and has given her a unique place in modern scholarship on these issues. What I hope this foreword will say to people, perhaps glancing at it in a bookshop or online or before sitting down to study it, is: "This is a book worth reading; it is engaged, passionate, and compassionate; it is a life-enhancing book about a phenomenon that ultimately does not afflict the gender minorities only, but us all, about the misunderstandings and prejudices that have bedevilled serious thought about the nature of that phenomenon and the consequences that such misunderstandings and prejudices still too often have".

John Harris FMedSci., FRSA., FSB., B.A., D.Phil., Hon.D.Litt.
Member *Academia Europaea*
Lord Alliance Professor of Bioethics
Director
Institute for Science, Ethics and Innovation
University of Manchester
Oxford Road
Manchester M13 9PL

Preface

And like all the most beautiful things, you lived one day only,
like a rose.

(*Marinella*, Fabrizio De André)[1]

When I was a teenager I happened to listen to the song whose final verses are quoted here. It is a poem in music written by the anarchic poet De André. The song is not about transgenderism. It narrates the story of a young woman (Marinella) who gently glides in a river in spring. The wind, admiring her beauty, embraces her and carries her over a star. The Prince, who loved her, will knock on her door to find her house empty and in despair will remain on her doorstep for a hundred years.

The poem is the romanced version of a real story. Marinella was the name of a seventeen-year-old girl, daughter of farmers, who became an orphan and was left without a home. She thus became a prostitute in order to survive. Two years later a client robbed her, killed her, and threw her body in the river Tanaro, in Italy.

"When I read this story on a local newspaper", De André narrates, "I had the impulse of doing something for her, in the only way I could [. . .] Given that I could no longer change her life for her, I decided to change her death, and I wrote this text as a sort of redemption, like in a fairy tale".

Marinella is thus the real story of a prostitute, brutally killed. It is a terrifying portrait of a secondary, humble character, mercilessly used, and not treated as a human being. It is an exceptional and indispensable story of a pariah, at the borders of humanity, at the limits of subordination.

Not only does the poem return her dignity, but, by honouring her beauty, it pays homage to her death.

For reasons that will become clearer in the course of this book, many transsexuals also end up in the street. Often discriminated against in their social life since childhood, disadvantaged in their employment, and sometimes alienated from healthcare services, transgender people sometimes find acceptance amongst peers and work as prostitutes. This may allow them to raise money for the hormones that are needed for their adjustment or for privately paid surgery, especially if they are clandestine immigrants. This exposes them to a number of perils, ranging from healthcare problems (including emotional trauma) to abuse and violence. Sometimes people get entangled in the justice system, from which it is particularly difficult to escape. Common prejudice may suggest that everyone chooses their lifestyle, and if people opt for street life, so be it. But it cannot be claimed that these people choose risky lifestyles and willingly expose themselves to violence. Trans are often left without recourse, and "people without recourse are not free"[2]. It is in one sense true that there is rather little desert in virtue, and rather little fault in error.

This book is inspired by compassion for a group whose condition is often surrounded by misunderstanding and prejudice, and by the wish to bring back the dignity that is often violated in these youths, to return a drop of the glow that such diversity brings to humankind.

Acknowledgments

The people who have contributed, directly or indirectly, to this volume are innumerable. I am hugely indebted to all those transgenders who have wanted to talk to me and make me understand their stories. Thanks to Prof. Max Elstain for having introduced me to the issue of transgender children. Terry and Bernard Reed and the whole Gender Identity Research and Education Society (GIRES) have been constantly helpful over the years and have represented a great source of inspiration for me in many ways. Among the people from whom I learnt a great deal I should mention Mike Besser, Peter Lee, Wylie Hembree, Ieuan Huges, Henriette Dele-marre, Garry Warne, Petra De Sutter, Walter Meyer, Richard Green, Peter Clayton, Polly Carmichael, Domenico Di Ceglie, Caroline Brian, Norman Spack, and Russell Viner. Peggy Cohen-Kettenis has provided crucial help with the medical parts of my book, and her encouragement has been much appreciated. I am hugely grateful to Margaret Brazier and Nishat Hyder for helping with the legal parts, whose complexities have challenged me enormously. In addition to the preceding, I wish to thank John Harris and Simon Barnes for reading and commenting on my work. A special thanks goes to Dino Topi and Muireann Quigley, who have carefully read (and proofread) the whole manuscript and given extensive comments. My gratitude also goes to all my colleagues at the Centre for Social Ethics and Policy and at the Institute for Science Ethics and Innovation at the University of Manchester, and to the whole School of Law, which allowed time and support for me to complete this book.

Introduction

Brothers humans, who will live after us
Have no hardened hearts against us
Because if you have pity for us, poor
God will sooner have pity of you.
You see us here, hanging, five or six of us
And our flesh, too nourished
After a long time is devoured and putrid to the bone
We are dust and ash.
Of our misfortune nobody rejoice
But pray to God that he forgave us all!
Do not disdain it
If we call you Brothers
Even if we are killed by justice.
However you know how turbulent is a man's soul.
Forgive us because we have passed towards the Virgin Mary's son
That his grace be not arid
And he preserved us from the infernal flames.
We are dead, nobody tormented us
But pray to God that he absolved us all!
The rain has washed us enough
The sun has darkened and dried us
Magpies and crows have dug into our eyes
Pulled our beards and eyebrows.

Never, not one single moment, we remain seated
Here and there, as the wind, blowing at its ease does
Without a pause, we are tossed
And hit and pecked by the birds.
Do not join our confraternity
But pray to God that he absolved us all.
Prince Jesus, you have the power over all
Make it that the hell has no power on us: we have nothing to share
*   with it.*
Men, now, do not deride us
But pray to God that he absolved us all.

This poem was written in the 1400s by the French poet François Montcor-
bier, better known as François Villon. Villon was a *man of letters*; he
obtained a degree from the University of Paris and later a licence as a *maître*

dès arts still from Paris. One day Villon was caught in a fight where a priest died. Villon was arrested and subsequently released as it was found he acted in self-defence. Villon continued his life as a vagabond poet, continually caught in crimes and living at the margins of society.[1] From that 'edge', he could witness a reality, a section of humankind, of which he would have remained ignorant had he proceeded in his wealthy and comfortable life. From this new periphery, Villon acquired a different perspective on the human condition.

The poem cited in the preceding, known as the *Ballade des pendus* or the *Epitaph of Villon (L'épitaphe Villon)*, represents the last moments and the final words of a group of men condemned to death. It is thought that Villon wrote this poem while in prison, waiting to be executed.

In this poem, the men on death row walk through the crowd and exhort people to have compassion for them and for all human beings alike. It is the awareness of the frailty of human life that, the poem suggests, should ingrain compassion in those who observe. The poem is a declaration of equality of all human beings: nobody is truly innocent (*you know how turbulent is a man's soul*). The observers are in one sense in no better situation than the condemned (*God forgive us all*). Men on death row are thus an allegory of the human condition, constantly at the border of mistake and death.

In quoting this poem I am not of course comparing transsexualism to imprisonment or criminality. I compare, instead, trans groups to other marginalised and ostracised minorities. This poem is quoted also because it inspires us all to suspend judgment, and because it celebrates the value of understanding those who appear different: in the case of the poem, these are those accused and despised (rightly or wrongly); in our case, these are the gender minorities. The poem reminds us that we are all dangling before a common undulating, uncertain destiny, swaying between error, virtue, and fortune.

It is this awareness that compels us to rethink what happens to other people beyond the way in which their experiences are normally conceptualised, and thus to critically reflect, in our case, on what it is to experience 'Gender Identity Disorder', what this refers to, what life is like for children with this condition, how it is best to think about it, and how to approach what appears at a first sight as a curious and puzzling dis-ease[2] with what should be the smoothest aspect of one's growth, namely, gender.

At various times in this book, some anarchic poets and artists will also be cited. I will be unable to render justice to their contribution to culture; I will only use them to illustrate how minorities may be understood and celebrated. Various anarchic poets have celebrated the value of those who are different, in culture, race, or morals, and who are often discriminated against only for reasons relating to their difference, and sometimes turned themselves into one of them (like Villon). Some artists have questioned in very provocative ways the very notion of normality over which such discrimination is held. I will discuss some of the works of so called *Angels of anarchy*. As an allegory of the despised, sometimes the aesthetic beauty of the back corners is honoured. Majakovskij exhorts: *Fall in love under the sky of the brothels, with the poppies in the majolica milk jugs.*[3] Guccini will compare the beauty of a woman not to the exquisiteness of roses or orchids, but to *the flowers and the grass of the railways banks.*[4] De André will remind us that *nothing is born from diamonds, and from manure, flowers are born.*[5] The ordinary details, rarely honoured in arts or public discourses, become in some of these works the allegory of the people of no cast.

Stylistically, this book combines a rather technical analysis with the use of literary sources and fairy tales. Thus, a thorough clinical description of gender variance, theories of gender identity development, therapeutic strategies, and so on, will be provided. An ethical and legal analysis will follow: this is meant to address the main ethical and legal concerns that doctors may have while treating trans children, and that trans children and their families may have regarding their rights to access medical treatment. Although the analysis will be technical, fairy tales, quotes from poems and songs, and other literary images will be found as well as case histories. The reason is that I want to inspire the readers to think about gender minorities through various perspectives and not just as a clinical case.

There is a second and equally important reason why I mix various styles in this book: philosophers who, like me, have specialised in healthcare ethics, often mature a tendency to write books aimed at healthcare professionals or at other healthcare philosophers. But perhaps there is nothing that healthcare professionals should know, that sufferers, including children, should not also know. Gender concerns us all: we are all either men or women or a part of gender minorities. Indeed, I will suggest that we are all somehow *in between*, and a discourse of who we are and why we are who we are is one that should be of interest to everyone.

This book poses some simple questions: what is transgenderism, what happens to children who have 'atypical' gender development, and how should these children be helped? Although the questions are straightforward, the answers are complex, as they involve an understanding of what gender is, how it develops, and what 'normal' and 'atypical' gender identification are. In order to explore these more fundamental issues, it is necessary to recast our own ideas and perceptions around what it is to be a woman or a man, a girl or a boy. While exploring these more fundamental issues, it will become clear that some of the misunderstandings around transgenderism are rooted in philosophical doubts and debates that have a centuries-long history.

I will begin this book by setting the scene. In the first chapter I will talk about transsexualism generally, not just as it afflicts children, and explain what terms I use and why. In the second chapter, I begin the analysis of gender variance, and I start by attempting to offer an understanding of what 'gender' means. I then proceed in Chapter 3 to explain how gender identity is thought to develop, and various theories of gender identity development will be explained. In Chapter 4, I move to the exploration of transgenderism in children. I use case histories and clinical descriptions and I explore the various dimensions of this condition (the intra-psychic, the physical, and the social dimensions). After having done so, I give an account of the various therapies available, and, in Chapters 6 and 7, I explore the ethical and legal issues that such therapies may give raise to. In Chapter 8 I will pose a more general question relating to whether transgenderism is appropriately conceptualised as a mental illness, and I conclude that it is not. This leads me, in Chapter 9, to debate whether treatment should nonetheless be publicly funded. Chapter 10 contains a general conclusion. Some chapters will be longer than others; the reason is simply that there was sometimes more to say on one particular issue.

1 Transgenderism
Setting the Scene

1 INTRODUCTION

Far out in the ocean, where the water is very, very deep and as blue as the prettiest cornflower, and as clear as crystal, there dwells the Sea King. In his kingdom grow the most singular flowers and plants, and the fish swim happily. In the deepest spot of all stands the castle of the Sea King. Its walls are built of coral, the roof is made of shells, and the long windows are of the clearest amber. The Sea King had six beautiful daughters, but the youngest was the prettiest of them all. Her skin was as pale and delicate as a rose leaf, and her eyes as blue as the deepest sea; but, like all the others, she had no feet, and her body ended in a fish's tail. Their grandmother had promised each of them that they would be able to rise up out to the land when they would reach the age of fifteen. They would be able to watch the moonlight, to sit on the rocks and look at the large ships sailing on the sea surface, and could even see the towns and forests and all other wonders in the land of humans. The youngest mermaid still had five years to wait till she was allowed to go. One by one, her sisters had risen up and come down with the most extraordinary stories. Finally, the long-waited day arrived for the beautiful mermaid, and she rose up to the sea. As we all know, she fell in love with a Prince [. . .].

"I know what you want," said the sea witch. "It is very stupid of you, but you shall have your way, and it will bring you to sorrow, my pretty princess. You want to get rid of your fish's tail, and to have two supports instead of it, like human beings on earth, so that the young prince may fall in love with you". And then the witch laughed loud and disgustingly: "I will prepare a draught for you. Once you drink it, your tail will disappear and shrink up into what mankind calls legs, and you will feel great pain, as if a sword were passing through you. But all who see you will say that you are the prettiest little human being they ever saw. But at every step you take you will be in great pain; it will feel as if you were treading upon sharp knives [. . .]"

"I will bear with all that," said the little princess.

"But think again," said the witch. "For when once your shape has become like a human being, you can no more be a mermaid, and if the Prince will marry another woman, your heart will break, and you will become foam on the crest of the waves".[1]

The sad ending of the *Mermaid* is well known. The girl did not gain the love of the Prince, and she melted as foam of the ocean. She paid for wishing to become *whole*.

The Mermaid colourfully represents the unbearable discomfort that some people experience in living with the body they are given, and the price that some may have to pay in order to fulfil their desire to conform to whom they are. Interestingly, some sources suggest that Andersen was a transgender,[2] and that the Mermaid is an allegory of his being *in between*.

Whether or not Andersen was a transgender, and whether or not he consciously wanted to offer an illustration of transgenderism (or, more precisely, what is today called transgenderism), the Mermaid offers a poignant and beautiful literary representation of *being beyond birth*.

Gender ambiguity has not been central to children literature. A study by Weitzman et al.,[3] published in 1972, showed that the portrait of the two sexes in the literature for preschool children has typically been characterised by a rigid gender polarisation, with inflexible gender clichés, often discriminatory against the woman, and with little or no contemplation of genders going beyond the classic 'male'–'female' divide.[4] Later studies on the gender stereotypes in children education showed similar results.[5]

In 1995 the Council of Europe expressed the worry that such gender divide in children's literature may create models of behaviour that are penalising for women and that reinforce sexism. A 1995 Resolution invited the member states to promote a diversified image of women and men in society, in order to remove sexist and discriminatory messages from advertisements, media, and education.[6]

'Sexism' in this Resolution (coherently with typical usage) refers to discrimination *against women*. However, sexism may also affect those who are neither precisely men nor women, that is, the gender minorities, and even men (nailed by the same pin in prefixed roles).

The gender divide, with its rigid assignation of roles and responsibilities, has been at the centre of a heated debate regarding justice and equality between women and men. However, the rigid allocation of individuals to one gender or the other, with the overarching implications this has, affects the gender minorities as well. Being excluded by the equation, they suffer a perhaps even more profound discrimination.

Shrek, released in 2001, was probably the first cartoon[7] ever to have represented transgenderism. In *Shrek 2* (2004) the barwoman is a transgender (male to female) who is in love with a beautiful prince (a handsome man with some feminine traits—for example, he wears lipstick).[8] For the first time transgenderism is presented to children, regarded as normal and harmless.

The fact that transgenderism only recently made its appearance in children's literature is no great surprise. Transgenderism seems to be a relatively 'novel' medical condition, included in diagnostic manuals only since 1980 and still surrounded by copious contention relating to its features, causes, and outcome. Transgenderism is often associated, in common discourse, with deviant sexual behaviour, lust, and prostitution,[9] themes from which children, some may believe, should be protected. Many people ignore that children can be transgender and cannot easily make sense of what appears as a paradox.

However, transgenderism has contributed to popular culture and common imaginary, albeit in a symbolic way. Many traditional tales can be viewed as allegories of transgenderism: indeed, they *are* stories of transgenderism, if the word is understood in its etymological meaning. The Mermaid, Pinocchio, and many other tales are stories of children condemned by a joke of nature or by a magic spell to be different and marginalised only by reason of their difference. In many of these tales the redemption occurs when, by desert or fortune, fate changes and the protagonists finally become *physically similar to who they are*, when they *look like themselves*.

2 SETTING THE SCENE: THE 'DISCOVERY' OF TRANSSEXUALISM

It was only around the 1940s that David Cauldwell, an American psychologist, coined the word 'trans-sexual'. The word 'transgenderist' is attributed to Virginia Prince and dates much later (1987).[10] Since then, there has been a variety of attempts to produce terms that may capture appropriately the condition of gender minorities (see later in this chapter).[11] Many languages seem unable to refer to people who are neither *he* nor *she*, having only the masculine or feminine pronouns to indicate people and leaving thus the gender binary distinction intact at a linguistic level. This linguistic difficulty is sometimes taken as the reflection of a conceptual void: people in Western society cannot *think* of human beings that are neither men nor women, and thus lack a consistent language to refer to them.[12]

Cauldwell, after giving a name to the condition, began to recognise it as different from homosexuality, and as one needing clinical attention.[13] In doing so, he also initiated the process of medicalisation of gender variance. Lewins writes: "The substantial clinical literature on transsexualism has grown along with its increasing social visibility and claims that transsexuals 'are no longer regarded as freaks or perverts but as people with genuine problems deserving compassion, understanding, and appropriate medical and social management' (Walters and Ross 1986:ix)."[14]

Ten years after Cauldwell coined the term 'trans-sexual', Henry Benjamin, an American sexologist who became famous for his work with transsexuals, contributed to the acquisition of the term and to the awareness of this condition within the healthcare community.[15] This process of medicalisation, although it has had the benefit of allowing sufferers to be identified and receive specialised medical attention, has had its downfalls, which will be explored in Chapters 8 and 9. One of its pitfalls is that, by presenting transgenderism as pathology, with a date of birth and specific clinical features, it clouds the fact that this condition has (as somehow obvious) always been a part of human history.[16] No medical disadvantage is inherent to transgenderism, and different societies at different times have treated it in very diversified ways (for more, see Chapter 3, Section 9).

3   EARLY TRANS

There is a significant body of literature discussing the presence of transgenderism in the ancient past. Morris, in her seminal book *Conundrum*, writes:

> God, said the Jewish chronicler, created man in his own androgynous image—'male and female created he them', for in him both were united. Mohammed on his second coming, says the Islamic legend, will be born of a male. Among Christians, Paul assured the erring Galatians, there was no such thing as male or female—'all one person in Christ Jesus'.
>
> The Hindu pantheon is frequented by male–female divinities, and Greek mythology too is full of sexual equivocations, expressed in those divine figures who, embracing in themselves strength and tenderness, pride and softness, violence and grace, magnificently combine all that we think of as masculine or feminine.
>
> [. . .] The Phrygians of Anatolia [. . .] castrated men who felt themselves to be female, allowing them henceforth to live in the female role, and Juvenal, surveying some of his own fellow-citizens, thought the same plan might be adopted in Rome. [. . .] Hippocrates reported the existence of 'un-men' among the Scythians: they bore themselves as women, did women's work, and were generally believed to have been feminized by divine intervention. In ancient Alexandria we read of men 'not ashamed to employ every device to change artificially their male nature into female'—even to amputation of their male parts.[17]

The Night, sculpted by Michelangelo,[18] represents someone with both male and female attributes. The *Night* has manly thighs and womanly breasts, and it is not clear whether it is a man or a woman.[19] Gender ambiguity is here pictured as nearly a dreamy state.

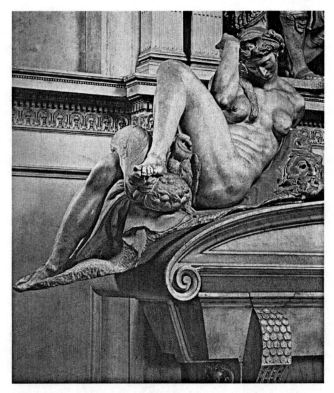

Figure 1.1   The Night by Michelangelo Buonarroti.

As we shall see in Chapter 3, different societies at different times have responded in a variety of ways to the presence of people who are neither males nor females: in many societies, their presence has been and is validated and valued. Although gender ambiguity has always been a part of human history, arts, and mythology, Western societies have failed to recognise the condition until the last century, and Western medicine has been caught unprepared to provide medical help to those who need it to deal with the discordance between their perceived gender identity and their apparent sex characteristics.

Jan Morris, who sought assistance for gender transition in the 1950s, tells us of expensive and fruitless trips to Harley Street in London, visiting psychiatrists and sexologists: "None of them—she wrote—knew anything about the matter at all, though none of them admitted it [. . .] Could it not be, they sometimes asked, that I was merely a transvestite, a person who gained a sexual pleasure from wearing the clothes of the opposite sex, and would not a little harmless indulgence in that practice satisfy my, er, somewhat indeterminate compulsion? Alternatively, was I sure that I was not just a suppressed homosexual, like so many others?"[20]

In an interesting essay, Hekma explains the way in which transsexual-ism was originally related to sexual deviance and homosexuality.[21]

Although as a 'condition', transsexualism appeared only in the 1950s, there have been many recorded cases of people who secretly passed to the other gender by cross dressing, and lived in the other gender, sometimes undiscovered until after their death.[22] Some of these were treated clinically even during the first decades of the 1900s.

Amongst the known cases, Alan L. Hart (1890–1962) is one of the earli-est female to male trans. Born as Alberta Lucille Hart, he took the name of Alan, and dressed and lived as a man before having any surgery. He gradu-ated in Oregon as a doctor and married a woman in 1918. In the same year he had hysterectomy.. Living as a trans man in the medical profession led Alan to many deceptions and changes of house and jobs.[23]

Lily Elbe, born Einar Mogens Wegener in Denmark, is another of the known earliest trans. She was a male to female transsexual. She underwent surgery in Berlin in 1930. It is thought that she wanted to have children, and had ovarian and uterine tissue implanted. She died, it is believed, as a result of this operation.[24]

Another early trans was Michael Dillon (1915–1960), born Laura, a female to male transsexual. Being a young trans university student, already living as Michael before surgery, he was struck by the knowledge of the developments of plastic surgery after the war. He heard that plastic sur-geons were now able to reconstruct the genitals of soldiers who had been injured during the war, and persuaded Sir Harol Gillies, Britain's top plas-tic surgeon, to build a penis for him. Several operations were carried out to this purpose, between 1946 and 1949.

Another case is that of Roberta (originally Robert) Cowell, a male to female trans.[25] After working as a pilot, being a prisoner of war and a motor racing driver, and marrying and having two children, Robert grew persuaded that he was repressing his feminine side, and after extensive psy-chotherapy he underwent surgery and became Roberta.

Between 1952 and 1954 George Jorgensen also had surgery and became Christine. Another well known case is that of April Ashley, who transi-tioned in 1960. Her case is famous because of the legal battle she endured. In 1963 she married Arthur Cameron Corbett. After fourteen days, Arthur decided to end the marriage and pleaded the courts to declare the marriage null by reason that April was of the male sex.[26] Even if she had had surgery, it was held that normal sexual intercourse could not take place with a com-pletely 'artificial cavity'. The precedent this set was finally turned around in the UK by the 2004 Gender Recognition Act.[27] This is an act of the Parliament of the United Kingdom, which gives people the right to change gender and establishes the way in which the various legal aspects of gender transition may take place. Importantly, the 2004 Gender Recognition Act does not require sex change surgery in order for transition to take place. In this way, the act effectively disconnects genital anatomy from gender identity, and recognises that people may have a gender identity that does not conform to their gender of assignment and to their genital anatomy.

The pioneering clinical work gave recognition to those people whose perceived gender did not match with their gender of assignment and rearing. Nonetheless, for a long time there has been wide confusion as to what the condition involved and how people should be treated. This confusion continues to surround transgenderism, especially in children and adolescents. Many people ask how it is possible for a child 'to know' that s/he is a trans; many ask whether this is an illness, and how this can be corrected. Even in clinical practice, as we are going to see in this book, there is wide disagreement regarding what the condition is, how it should be understood, what the treatment goals should be, and how these can appropriately be achieved.

Refining our understanding of transgenderism in children is crucial in order to define clearer clinical and ethically sound strategies of intervention. But before attempting to unravel what transgenderism is, it is necessary to try to disentangle the complexities inherent to the very notion of gender. As Raymond rightly points out, "transsexualism goes to the question of what gender is, how to challenge it, and what reinforces gender stereotyping in a role-defined society".[28]

As we shall see, no univocal answer can be provided to the question of what gender is. Gender is an elusive notion, with the chameleonic property of acquiring different meanings in different research contexts and disciplines. The analysis of the notion of gender within different contexts, and of the various theories of gender identity development, will all gesture towards the conclusion that there is not *one normal* type and *one abnormal* or disordered type of gender identity development. The clinical and normative implications that this may have will be discussed in the book.

I will conclude this chapter by offering some terminological clarifications.

4 TRANSWHAT?

The understanding and definition of transgenderism raises innumerable controversies and debates. Broadly speaking, transgenderism refers to the mismatch between assigned and perceived gender (in Chapter 4 I will discuss the condition, as it appears in children). However, some sources differentiate *transgenderism* from *transsexualism*, and the differentiation is itself open to debate. According to some, *transgenderism* refers to those who simply experience a mismatch between sense of gender and assigned gender, whereas *transsexualism* refers to those who take some steps in order to conform their bodies to their experienced gender, with, for example, hormonal treatment, dressing, or even surgery;[29] according to others, instead, *transsexuals* are those who have cross sex surgery, whereas all others are *transgender*.[30] Whether *transgender* should be used rather than *transgender*ed may be another matter of controversy. The use of the *dash* raises further problems:

should it be *trans-sexuals* or just *transsexuals*? And if the noun is used for *transsexual* why couldn't *transgender* also be used as a noun (thus with the plural *transgenders*, rather than *transgender [or trans-gender, or transgendered, or trans-gendered]* people)? Things become even more complicated when one considers transvestites, those who cross genders but not permanently and without medical aids but only with 'cosmetic' and removable aids (which of course raises the issue of how we should differentiate between medical and nonmedical aids), and who typically claim to belong to the gender of assignment (although nonsurgical transgender may also cross genders intermittently), and homosexuals, who do not feel as though they belong to the other gender but may indeed be very effeminate men or very masculine women (thus somewhat crossing the gender boundaries). Someone has used the term "pansexual"[31] to describe those who are not 'trans'itioning but who embrace various facets of both genders. If we consider the controversies surrounding the psychiatric nosology, the matter further entangles itself: as we shall see in Chapter 4, currently transsexualism is classified in diagnostic manuals as 'Gender Identity Disorder' (GID), but some have contested that transsexualism is not a disorder, and Domenico Di Ceglie coined the term 'Atypical Gender Identity Organisation' (AGIO).[32]

To make things sufficiently easy and avoid further confusion, in this book I will not differentiate between *transsexualism* and *transgenderism* (without denying that there are differences in the ways in which trans—or transvestites, or homosexuals, or, for what matters, heterosexuals—experience their gender and sexual orientation). I will also use *transgender* as a noun as well as an adjective. Thus, I may refer to *a transgender* as I may refer to *a transsexual*: I will use *transgender child* but I will also use *transgender* on its own as a noun. I will avoid transgender*ed* because grammatically it is incorrect as it would be incorrect to say *transsexualed*, although I respect other authors' choices on the matter. For the purposes of this book, the use of the dash is irrelevant, so I will go for transsexual and transgender rather than trans-sexual and trans-gender. In this context, what is relevant is the recognition that there are many different ways in which gender identity may develop, and thus "multiple social identities".[33] Although I am aware that some in the trans community may be keen to differentiate themselves from homosexuals and transvestites, I will group all those identities together, and I will use the terms *transgender, gender minorities, gender nomads, people with gender variance, atypical gender,* and *transsexuals* interchangeably.

Although I will use all those terms, I tend generally to privilege the word *transgender* because its etymological meaning captures what is mainly at stake in this book. *Transgender* etymologically means *beyond (trans) birth (gender)*, and this embraces all forms of development that are found in gender minorities. In addition to its aesthetic beauty, this term encompasses the existence and equal legitimacy of all forms of development that go beyond what is expected at birth.

Considering gender minorities as people who have gone *beyond birth* (rather than people who, say, use surgery) sets the bar of transgenderism very low. From this point of view, one does not need to have had hormones or any medical treatment to be transgender. Therefore, my terminology, it may be objected, may be 'all inclusive'. Whereas this is true, this is not a limit. Understanding transgenderism in this way allows us to think about the condition as one of the many ways in which people may recognise themselves as being different from what may be expected of them, for reason of birth or for reason of belonging to a certain race, or social class, or ethnic class, or culture. In this wider sense, transgenderism is on a continuum line with the condition of anyone who may seek to live a life that is authentic to themselves as individuals. Viewing transgenderism not as a phenomenon standing on its own, but as one of the many ways in which people may place themselves beyond any stated border in the attempt to live up to who they think and feel they are, has the important advantage of allowing a better understanding of the condition. It gives a key to anyone, whether or not experiencing gender dysphoria, to understand this phenomenon as one of the many ways in which people may refuse authorities (be they explicit or implicit) in which they do not recognise themselves and search a more authentic life for themselves. It also allows us to distract the attention from a discourse on the role that *genitals* play in this phenomenon, as the condition is often misguidedly portrayed as genital dysmorphism, and therefore allows an understanding of the more profound meaning that transgenderism may have for the individual concerned, and perhaps for society at large. Setting transgenderism in this guise should finally allow us to disclose the value added to humankind of this, like of other, form of transitioning and diversity.

5 CONCLUSIONS

In this chapter I have offered a brief history of this condition and some terminological clarifications.

In this book, as the title suggests, I am mainly concerned with transgenderism in children and adolescents.[34] However, in this chapter I have sketched some of the hurdles relating to transgenderism more generally. This chapter has set the scene, by illustrating some of the complexities implicated in transgenderism and some of the tensions in the way one may think about it.

This book proposes a way of understanding transgenderism in young people and a way of thinking about how to best deal with their suffering. But in order to do this, it is preliminarily necessary to explore the notions of gender and gender identity and understand how gender identity development is thought to occur.

This book suggests that gender variance is not a disorder or an anomaly. This is so for two reasons: one is that the assumption that, from a biological point of view, there are two sexes and two genders, and what departs from this is pathological, is a value laden interpretation of a much more complex array of facts. The critique of gender norms, mainly prompted by feminist intellectuals and artists, inspired an important change in common morality and in the ordinary way we think about men and women, and their respective social roles (see Chapter 2). But sex can and should also be deconstructed. The idea that in 'nature' only two sexes are present, and that whatever differs is pathology, is misguiding, and this has important conceptual and normative implications in the way transgenderism may be understood and dealt with.

The other reason is that, as I will argue, gender identity cannot develop in a predictable way in any case. This implies that there is not one normal and one abnormal way of developing: gender development is a complex and scarcely understood process in all cases. But in order to clarify all this, it is preliminarily necessary to explain what gender and gender identity are.

2 What Is Gender?

Man is double. There are two beings in him: an individual being
which has its foundation in the organism [...] and a social being
[...] In so far as he belongs to society, the individual transcends
himself, both when he thinks and when he acts.

(Emile Durkheim, 1912) [1]

1 INTRODUCTION

Originally 'gender' was a philosophical notion, indicating a category of
objects that have some essential properties in common. A clear definition of
the term, in its logical meaning, was provided by Aristotle: "Gender is what
is predicated according to the essence of many which differ specifically". [2]
For example, in the definition of 'man' as a 'rational animal', animal indicates gender, whereas rational expresses the specific difference. Discourses
on gender encompassed ontological speculations: in Plato gender is a "note
of the real" (for example, in the *Sophist* 253*d*), [3] and he distinguished five
genders: being, movement, quiet, identity, and diversity. Aristotle did not
consider gender as the substance, but as one of the necessary attributes
of the substance, and, in the *Categories* (5,2*b*) he talked about gender as
"second substance". [4] The Sophists, in the fifth century BC used the notion
of gender "to describe the threefold classification of the names of things as
masculine, feminine, and intermediate". [5] In contemporary logic, gender is
not used in an ontological sense, and it denotes a category that includes a
variety of subcategories.

Gayle Rubin, in *The Traffic in Women*, has used the notion of *gender* to
denote the meanings that societies attribute to sexed bodies. [6] Gender from
now onward becomes a more "politically correct" [7] way to refer to 'sex', and
alludes to the interpretation given to the biological facts in certain cultural
and social contexts. Thus gender has somehow reacquired the substantive
original flavour: it is used to somehow define the sort of being that one is.

However, in this translation from logic to ontology, the notion has also
assumed very blurred boundaries, and its meaning has lost the original
definition. It is, in fact, now used in remarkably different ways in different
contexts, and for this reason, it can be hard to reconcile the various ways in
which gender may be understood.

This chapter will provide an account of various ways in which gender
and gender identity are interpreted, in disciplines such as sociology and
gender studies, on the one hand, and in supposedly more scientific disciplines such as psychiatry and endocrinology, on the other. I will also offer

some reflections on the philosophical underpinnings and background of these notions. A brief history of philosophy is important to appreciate the deeper meanings that these widely used and scarcely understood notions may have.

2   GENDER IN DIFFERENT DISCOURSES: IN SOCIOLOGY AND FEMINIST/GENDER STUDIES

The vast literature on gender and Gender Identity Disorder (GID) shows that the notion of gender has different meanings in different contexts.

In sociology and feminist/gender studies,[8] the term *gender* is usually associated with the roles that an individual has in a given context or system (family or society). *Gender identity* refers to the perception that one person has of her/himself, of her/his belonging to a biological sex, of her/his roles within various systems. Gender identity is the recognition of the implications of belonging to one sex.[9] The roles, behaviours, and attitudes that people may adopt and internalise, depending on whether they belong to one sex or another, reflect the expectations that a society in a given historical and geographical context has of men and women.

The construction of gender identity begins at birth or even before, when the parents become aware of the sex of the child. Based on this acknowledgment, various learning experiences for the child begin to be gender biased. Genitals are thought to reveal a series of relationships, preferences, and inclinations, which are assumed to be stable across the future life of the child. We will get back later to the studies that indicate how parental behaviour 'shapes' gender identity (see Chapter 3).

The common denominator of sociological and gender studies is that many features of gender are the result of implicit and/or explicit social and cultural norms. Gender is a social and political construct, and it reflects normative ideas of how society should be organised. In a given society, individuals must continually testify their gender belonging through language, behaviour, and social roles. The concepts of 'man' and 'woman' are dynamic, and must be understood in the specific historical, geographical, and cultural context. It is society that determines what it is to be man or woman.[10]

Gender studies oppose the idea that the classification of genders is purely biologically determined and denounce the social consequences that this has had, in particular for women. 'Naturalistic', 'biological', or 'essentialist' claims (such as women are 'empathic and nurturing' by nature and therefore they are 'by nature' best suited for childrearing) have a precise political significance: these claims are, or can be, forces of social and political oppression.

As Lewins writes:

> The assumption that gender differences are somehow the result of biological sex differences has been largely discredited by a substantial

body of literature. There is a growing tide of academic opinion that supports the idea that gender is constructed in a social context and can even be chosen instead of gender dichotomy being 'forced upon us by nature' [. . .] The social construction of gender is corroborated by the principal insights of anthropologists who have scrutinised gender from a cross cultural perspective [. . .] cross cultural research on gender reveals ways of attributing gender other than biological sex differences and the non universality of two genders. In terms of transsexualism, this literature helps challenge the taken for granted link of sex and gender and [. . .] seriously challenge the assumption thematic in the clinical approach that transsexualism is pathology.[11]

According to this view, not only is the notion of gender a social construct, but also *transsexualism*. "Transsexualism seems to exist primarily as a result of gender dimorphism on the part of society"[12]. Gender studies thus criticise biological determinism. They stress how the construct of the concepts of 'man' and 'woman' (and thus *transsexual*) are *relational*, rather than biological.[13] This has precise social, ethical, and political implications, as we shall see in the next sections.

Gender studies also differentiate between 'sex' and 'gender'. Sex is often taken to refer to the sum of the biological traits that produce a phenotype. Sex refers to the genetic and chromosomal makeup of an individual, to the anatomy and the physiology of the individual. In simple terms, 'sex' refers to four biological facts: chromosomes, gonads, hormones, and physical appearance. However, as we are now going to see, the differentiation between sex and gender is not as straightforward as it is sometimes assumed. Even the 'biological facts' are not just *facts* but interpretations, perhaps resulting from assumptions relating to what human 'nature' should be (see the following). I will show that this has wide ranging implications for the way transgenderism should be understood. But in order to capture all this, it is first necessary to understand the way sex and gender are differentiated.

2.1 The 'Biological' Sex

A significant part of the literature on gender (including the literature which criticises biological determinism) differentiates between *sex and gender*. This, I will argue here, is problematic and may have significant negative implications in terms of the way transgenderism is understood and treated.

Sex is thought to refer to a number of biological 'facts'. Thus sex is typically defined as follows:

First there is the 'chromosomal sex' (XX; XY); the twenty-third pair of chromosomes determines chromosomal sex. In cases in which the chromosomes are both XX the embryo generally will become female;

in cases in which the chromosomes are XY, the embryo generally will become male. Sex differentiation begins to occur around the sixth week of gestation. Until then, all embryos are sexually undifferentiated, although the basic structure is female.

At this stage we have the expression of so called 'gonadal sex' (testicles and ovaries are the primary anatomical sex characteristics, which are often a function of chromosomal sex). Typically, at week six to eight, the embryo develops testicles (in the presence of a Y chromosome) or ovaries (in the presence of an X chromosome). Once the testicles are formed, they produce androgen hormones, which contribute to the formation of the male internal and external organs.

This is the stage of 'hormonal sex', which induces differentiation at the second month of foetal life. If the levels of hormones produced are low or if, due to other anatomical characteristics, the embryo is insensitive to the androgen hormones, the embryo will continue to develop female characteristics. Therefore, in absence of a certain type of "chromosomal or hormonal information, the morphogenesis and subsequent development, at least for mammals, proceed spontaneously in the female direction".[14]

Lastly, there is the 'anatomical sex', which refers both to the internal reproductive organs and external phenotypical appearance (genitalia).[15]

Sometimes 'legal sex' is added to the list. Governmental agencies generally differentiate human beings as males and females, on birth certificates, driving licences, and other official documents. Human sexuality is thus typically regarded as dimorphic (*di = two; morph = type*).[16]

These briefly sketched here are the 'facts' that are thought to determine the 'sex' of an individual. Gender and gender identity are considered as the "social interpretation"[17] of these biological facts. Gender, in this meaning, is a social construct that applies to biological sex.

Things are not so simple, however. In addition to the X and Y chromosome, there seem to be at least twelve others across the human genome governing sex differentiation.[18] In the 1990s a gene determining the differentiation of tissue into testis was identified within the Y chromosome. This gene was called SRY (sex determining region of the Y), also known as TDF (testis development factor). It is thought that the SRY triggers a pathway of other genes that cause the gonads to continue to develop into a male. However, the way in which the SRY functions is not fully understood: in fact, there are SRY negative individuals who have testicles and SRY positive individuals who do not have testicles. In these latter cases, there seems to be another gene (this time within the X chromosome) called DAX-1, which can override the effects of the SRY, "so that an individual with XY chromosomes and a functioning SRY gene develops ovaries and not testes".[19] Other genes in other chromosomes, in addition to these, are also involved in sex differentiation: for example, the SF-1 on chromosome 9, the WR-1 on chromosome 11, the SOX-9 on chromosome 17, and MIS on chromosome 19.[20] The more sexual differentiation becomes unravelled, the more complex it appears, and the more it becomes clear that the classification reported in the preceding (including the classification of humans into males and females) is a simplification of a much more complex set of facts.

Another indication of the complexity of sex differentiation is the fact that in many cases the various aspects of sex differentiation are not congruent.[21] This can happen in humans as well as in other mammalians. Various hypotheses relating to the relationship between such incongruence and sexual behaviours in mammalians have been formulated, especially by behavioural endocrinologists, based on observations of nonhuman animals.[22] In humans there are conditions in which the various elements of sex do not combine with each other in the way I sketched here. For example, XY individuals could have external phenotypical appearances as women, and could be raised and identify themselves as women and the other way round.[23] These conditions are called *intersex conditions* or Disorders of Sex Development (DSDs).

2.2   Intersex: Disorders of Sex Development

Intermediate sexes were noted a long time ago. In 1030 Avicenna, an Arabian physician and philosopher, and author of the *Canon of Medicine*, provided one of the very first observations of intersex:

> Illi qui est hermaphroditus non est membrum viri, neque membrum mulieris, Et de illis est qui habet utrumque, sed unum eorum est occultius, et debilius, et aliud est e contrario: et egreditur urina ex uno eorum absque altero. Et de illis est in quo ambo sunt aequalia, et pervenit ad me, quod de illis est qui agit et patitur, sed parum verificatur hoc, Et multoties curantur per incisionem membri occultioris, et regimine vulneris eius.[24]

> (Those who are hermaphrodite possess neither the virile member nor the feminine member. And among them there are those who have both the one and the other, but one of them is more hidden and feeble, and the other is the opposite: and urine comes out of one of them but not the other. And among them, there are those who have both [members] equal [in dimension] and to my knowledge there are among them those who are active and those who are passive, but this is scarcely verified.[25])

Here Avicenna says that the hermaphrodite is the person who has neither the female nor the male member. Avicenna gave a medical classification of the phenomenon as well as medical recommendations.

The most common DSDs are Turner syndrome, Klinefelter syndrome, congenital adrenal hyperplasia (CAH), androgen insensitivity syndrome

(AIS), and 5-Alpha Reductase Deficiency. It should be noted that in many cases there is no medical complication associated with these conditions.

Turner syndrome affects females only and consists of an alteration of one of the sex chromosomes. Whereas people normally have two sex chromosomes, and females have two XX chromosomes, girls with the Turner syndrome have (most often) only one X chromosome.

Klinefelter syndrome is a condition characterised by the presence of one extra Y. Klinefelter syndrome is sometimes asymptomatic, but in some cases males may experience breast growth and have small testes; in females, reduced breast and ovaries size may be found.[26]

CAH concerns those enzymes that are responsible for processing steroids into sex hormones. As a result of an enzymatic variation, steroids become testosterone. The result is masculine appearance of the external genitalia. The level of masculinisation is variable and ranges from an enlargement of the clitoris to the appearance of a small penis. The internal organs are in these cases normal (ovaries, vagina, and uterus).

In AIS the individual who has XY sex chromosomes does not respond to androgens. People with AIS have genitalia that can look typically female in appearance (complete AIS or C-AIS) or ambiguous with features that range from typical male like to typical female like (partial AIS or P-AIS). Tissue response to oestrogen is present and breast development and other signs of feminisation occur. Female internal reproductive organs are missing or vestigial, and Wolffian duct derivatives (urogenital structures) persist. No relation between gene mutation and phenotype has been discovered. Infertility is common.[27]

5-Alpha Reductase Deficiency is a genetic condition that affects males only. A gene mutation causes what is in effect an intersex appearance. Biological males affected develop primary sex characteristics of females but have male gonads, including testicles and Wolffian structures.

2.3   The Relationship between Sex and Gender: Should It Be the Other Way Round?

When in literature gender is presented as the social interpretation of the biological facts, sex is presented as an observable datum, resulting from a clear set of biological markers. These biological markers are thought to differentiate animals in females and males, and human animals are no exception to this rule.

However, as the preceding section has shown, we know of a much more colourful and complex picture when it comes to sex differentiation. Saying that sex develops only in two ways is a simplification of a much more complex scenario.

It could be argued that these other types of sex development are pathological. But it is not clear why they should be regarded as pathological. Observation of sexual differentiation, as we have just seen, shows that there are *not* two sexes, but many more than two, depending on the way in which chromosomes, enzymes, and hormones work in each individual. If one had to remain faithful to the facts, one would have to conclude that there are not just two but several sexes in humans. As the geneticist Anne Fausto-Sterling argues, "biologically speaking, there are many gradations running from female to male; and depending on how one calls the shots, one can argue that along that spectrum lie at least five sexes—and perhaps even more".[28] The Intersex Society of North America also reports:

Intersex isn't a discreet or natural category [. . .]. Intersex is a socially constructed category that reflects real biological variation. [. . .] [N]ature presents us with sex anatomy spectrums. Breasts, penises, clitorises, scrotums, labia, gonads—all of these vary in size and shape and morphology. So-called 'sex' chromosomes can vary quite a bit, too. But in human cultures, sex categories get simplified into male, female, and sometimes intersex, in order to simplify social interactions, express what we know and feel, and maintain order. So nature doesn't decide where the category of 'male' ends and the category of 'intersex' begins, or where the category of 'intersex' ends and the category of 'female' begins. Humans decide [29].

To say that only two sexes are 'natural' or 'biologically appropriate', and that all others are pathological, seems to reveal the assumption of normative categories through which the biological 'facts' are interpreted. If we ask ourselves where biology got the idea that there are only two sexes, given that empirical evidence shows otherwise, and where it got the idea that some sexes are 'normal' and others are 'pathological', the normative assumptions begin to become explicit.

One answer, according to Herdt, may be found in Darwin's evolutionism. Herdt explains how the dogma of the two sexes as the 'biological norm' relates closely to Darwin's evolutionism and to the proposition that traits that are 'normal' are those that are functional to reproduction. According to Herdt, sexual dimorphism is meant to refer to the phylogenetically inherited structure, which, in evolutionary terms, is functional to those purposes. Thus "dimorphism reveals a deeper stress on 'reproduction' as a paradigm of science and society".[30] "Because male and female are tantamount to natural categories [. . .] it follows that the intermediate is unnatural, inverted or perverse".[31]

What is 'reproductive', however, is also culturally bound, and is thus not an 'observable datum'. Herdt, for example, cites some instances of societies in which what is reproductive is different from the Western idea of chromosomes and hormones. Men in Sambia, for example, inseminate boys in order to make them "reproductively competent".[32] Of course, this could be viewed as a symbolic enablement, but it is not clear how, in any given culture, symbolic and 'real' forms of reproductive abilities can be differentiated. For example, in spite of the stress on reproductive abilities as markers for sexual differentiation, postmenopausal women (who no longer have that ability) or otherwise infertile women or men are still regarded as females or males, and in this sense reproductive abilities can also be considered as symbolic. More importantly, the choice of 'being functional to reproduction' as a test for biological classification is to some extent arbitrary and sets out a 'biological norm' that leads to pathologising other forms of sexual development that are not inherently harmful or disadvantageous for the individual.

As we have seen earlier in this chapter, the various 'sex' elements are not always congruent. Sex is a complex set of occurrences. By arguing that *gender* is the process of social construction of biological features, gender studies seem to assume that the biological features are well identifiable and observable facts. The postulate here appears to be that biologically there are clear physical differences in humans and that there are well defined biological categories to which social and cultural *meanings* are historically attached. It seems instead that the very classification of sexes into males, females, and disorders depends on an implicit norm of functioning, which is based on gender norms. Therefore, perhaps the biological classification of sexes can be best understood by reversing the relationship between sex and gender: rather than seeing gender as a construction based on biological sex, we should perhaps think of sex (the dichotomous sex) as a construction based on implicit norms relating to gender (see Box 2.1).[33]

The very biological facts that should provide the 'substrate' for social constructs are themselves a matter of interpretation and construct, to an important extent, which cannot be separated from the social and cultural values of the observers. The biological classification of two sexes, and the dichotomy of sex and gender, thus, "is probably culturally bound and scientifically misleading".[34]

Box 2.1 Relationship between Gender and Sex				
Human societies	———▶	Gender as a form of social differentiation	———▶	The interpretation of observable facts in terms of sex differentiation
	Produce		Leads to	

Box 2.2   How Many People Are Affected by Disorders of Sexual Differentiation[35]

Not XX and not XY: one in 1,666 births.

Klinefelter (XXY): one in 1,000 births.

AIS: one in 13,000 births.

P-AIS: one in 130,000 births.

Classical CAH: one in 13,000 births.

Late onset adrenal hyperplasia: one in 66 individuals.

Vaginal agenesis: one in 6,000 births.

Ovotestes: one in 83,000 births.

Idiopathic (no discernable medical cause): one in 110,000 births.

Iatrogenic (caused by medical treatment, for instance, progestin administered to pregnant mother): no estimate.

5-Alpha Reductase Deficiency: no estimate.

Mixed gonadal dysgenesis: no estimate.

Complete gonadal dysgenesis: one in 150,000 births.

Hypospadias (urethral opening in perineum or along penile shaft): one in 2,000 births.

Hypospadias (urethral opening between corona and tip of glans penis): one in 770 births.

Total number of people whose bodies differ from standard male or female: one in 100 births.

Total number of people receiving surgery to "normalise" genital appearance: one or two in 1,000 births.

One further observation needs to be made in relation to gender studies: by emphasising the 'mouldable' character of gender, gender studies have suggested that gender is something that can be changed depending on the way parents, educators, and various actors behave with children at a developmental stage. Thus the authors of the child's future have the power to write a gendered script that is amenable to the interpretation of the author. The clinical implications this has had will be discussed later (see Chapter 3).

3   BACKGROUND: THE CRITIQUE OF SOCIAL INSTITUTIONS

Let us now return to the critique, addressed by gender studies, of the gender divide. This critique has important implications at several levels: psychological (gender studies question the way gender develops and the importance of genetic and chromosomal factors); philosophical (they question concepts and acquired notions); ethical (they insist on equal opportunities and rights against explicit or implicit forms of sex based discrimination); and political and social (they question the fabric of society as a whole, which is constructed upon the gender divide, with its political, social, and economic meanings).

The critique generally points to the fact that the gender binary distinction is not just descriptive, but hierarchical and therefore normative.[36] The category of men is superior to that of women. By virtue of allegedly 'natural' features, the woman is relegated to roles decided for her, and thus discriminated against. Her opportunities to participate in social life outside the family are restricted, 'based on nature'. The critique of sexism thus has larger implications relating to the organisation of institutions such as the modern family and relating to the whole capitalistic society.

Some of the works by various philosophers, in particular of the 1700s and 1800s, constitute the background for the debate on the meanings of gender identity and gender roles. Gender division and, in particular, reference to nature to determine the role of the woman in the fabric of society, are recurrent themes in the literature of the Enlightenment. Pierre Russel (1742–1802), for example, published a book called *Système physique et moral de la Femme* (Paris 1775). Here he tried to demonstrate that biology determines differences in characters between males and females, and this explains their different social roles. Cabanis, another French physician and philosopher, in his *Rapports du physique et du moral de l'homme* (Paris 1805), argued that all the differences between women and men were stemmed from women's physical weakness.

§ II

La faiblesse musculaire porte les femmes à des habitudes sédentaires, et à des soins plus délicats: les hommes ont besoin de plus de mouvement et d'un plus grand exercice de leur vigueur.

(The muscular weakness leads women to sedentary habits, and they are more delicate: men need more movement and greater exercise of their vigour.)

§ IV.

Chez les femmes, la pulpe cérébrale est plus molle, et le tissu cellulaire plus muqueux et plus lâche; tandis que chez les honmes, la vigueur du système nerveux et celle du système musculaire s'accroissent l'une par l'autre.

(In women, the cerebral mass is softer, and the cellular tissue more mucous and more lax; while in men, the vigour of the nervous system and that of the muscular system increase one another.[37])

Even Voltaire, who had always been very keen to discredit the traditional spiritualistic idea of the relation between sexes as god given, ended up with condemning women (and men) to the 'superior authority of nature'. In *Femmes, soyez soumises a vos maris*,[38] while stating that matrimony (with what we would call today *its gender roles*) is *a contract* chosen by the parties, and that therefore it is only valid insofar as it is based on equality and freedom, he argued that the woman's weakness determines her roles (and hence, the roles of the man): *her physique is the measure of her morality*. Hegel, mostly known for his theoretical studies of phenomenology and logic, in his *The Philosophy of Right*, argued that in the family "the woman has her substantial destination".[39]

During the Enlightenment, theoretical ideals of equality, free consensus, and civil contracts spread amongst intellectuals. Nonetheless, recurrent recourse to nature nailed women (as well as men) into fixed roles.

Also the father of Positivism, and the one who coined the term 'sociology', August Comte (1798–1857) believed that nature shapes social roles[40] (see also Chapter 3). 'Natural' differences determine social differences. Thus, for Comte, *a woman is born as a woman, does not become a woman*. Of course, a few decades later, as is well known, Simone de Beauvoir declared the opposite, that a woman *becomes a woman, and is not born as such*.[41] Comte also distanced himself from his friend John Stuart Mill (1806–1873), who strongly opposed any form of subjugation grounded on allegedly 'natural' factors.

Mill assimilated the subjection of women to the subjection of black people in America.[42] He brought to light the trap and dangers inherent in this shift to nature, which was used to justify and determine people's social roles. In *The Subjection of Women* he argued that appealing to nature in order to explain what roles people should have, and which family and social institutions are morally acceptable, is an apotheosis of instinct. This apotheosis of instinct is much sadder than the idolatry of rationality (which Mill found, for example, in Hegel and Kant). The apotheosis of instinct and nature supports the worst and most dangerous superstitions. Mill tried to demystify the concept of 'human nature' as a datum and immutable given fact. Biology, he pointed out, is one of the elements that shape human interactions, and it is in turn completed and shaped by equally important social and cultural facts. "What is now called the nature of women," Mill wrote, "is an eminently artificial thing".[43]

The demystification of the sacrality and immutability of the family is also an important part of the philosophical works of Marx and Engels.

3.1 Marx and Engels

Marx and Engels are mostly known for their contribution to the communist ideology, and Marx in particular for his reflection on Hegel's political thought. Yet both Marx and Engels have, more broadly, contested the fabric of society with its various institutions, here including the family. Marx and Engels highlighted the contradictions inherent in the capitalistic bourgeoisie society, and criticised not only the capitalistic economy with its social structure, but also the structure of the family and the condition of the woman, both within the family and within society. They considered the division of labour within the family as one of the pivots of the conservation of social relations in the capitalist economy and bulwark of the servitude of the woman.

In 1844 Marx and Engels published *The Holy Family*. They here refer to the "masterly characterisation of marriage"[44] made by Charles Fourier. Fourier, a socialist theorist, had contested the ill anomalies of modern social institutions, including the family, and argued that the degree of emancipation of women is the measure of the degree of general emancipation of a society.[45] Later, in 1884, in *The Origin of the Family, Private Property and the State*, Engels argued that the relationships that we know within a society (including the relationship between women and men, and their respective roles) are neither given by nature nor the produce of a teleological predefined or divine plan. Social institutions, such as the family, evolve historically and are influenced, in different ways, by economical forces.[46]

Engels had been profoundly influenced by the studies of Morgan, who applied the evolutionary criteria of Darwinism to the study of the family across time.[47] The nuclear, monogamist family, in which intimate cross generational relations are taboo (incest), is the product of evolution, Morgan argued. According to Engels, the differentiation of roles and powers between man and woman are contradictions, in the same way as capital and labour, city and countryside, working class and owners, among others. Quoting Marx, he wrote: "The modern family contains in germ not only slavery (servitus), but also serfdom, since from the beginning it is related to agricultural services. It contains in miniature all the contradictions which later extend throughout society and its state".[48]

Lenin (who did not write extensively about women's issues) also contributed to connecting the questions relating to the ethical legitimacy of the capitalist economy to the condition of the woman in the modern society.

> Present-day capitalist society conceals within itself numerous cases [of. . .] oppression which do not immediately strike the eye. [. . .] Millions upon millions of women [. . .] live (or, rather, exist) as 'domestic slaves'. It is these women that the capitalists most willingly employ as home-workers, who are prepared for a monstrously low wage to 'earn a little extra' for themselves and their family, for the sake of a crust of bread. It is from among these women, too, that the capitalists of all countries recruit for themselves (like the ancient slave-owners and the medieval feudal lords) any number of concubines at a most 'reasonable' price. And no amount of 'moral indignation' (hypocritical in 99 cases out of 100) about prostitution can do anything against this trade in

female flesh [. . .]. Slavery, feudalism and capitalism are identical in this respect. It is only the form of exploitation that changes; the exploitation itself remains.[49]

If social institutions (including the relationship between woman and man) are not given by nature or god, but are the result of a complex process of *becoming*, entirely based on material conditions (interrelationship of economic forces and social relations), it follows that these social institutions are not fixed and that they have no intrinsic normative value. They are amendable to review and criticism, as amendable to review and criticism as the other forms of polarisation that result from the modern economy.

The philosophical critique of division of labour between women and men (what we would now probably call *gender roles*) provided an important conceptual background for the social theories of gender development, which will be discussed Chapter 3.

Contemporary discussions about transgenderism replicate these older debates on the role of women in the family and society.[50] In trying to understand the causes of transgenderism, some have insisted on biological dysfunctions, some on upbringing, some on the intra-psychic problems of the sufferer. The answer to the question as to why some people do not fit in the assigned gender and the very way this question is posed have important implications for clinical practice. We will discuss this in Chapters 3, 4, and 5.

It is important to note that whereas the philosophical debates briefly outlined here concern the subjugation of *women* to assumptions relating to what is allegedly 'natural', in fact those allegedly 'natural' authorities also subjugate *men*. The authority of institutions that, based on 'biology' and therefore regarded as 'natural', becomes conceptually indisputable, compels everyone (not only women) into roles that may be fixed and immutable. This has a precise clinical significance when we come to deal with gender minorities. If in the gender divide the woman is placed in an 'inferior' class (the *second* sex, to use the words of Simone de Beauvoir), those who are neither women nor men, or who are gender nomadic, who cross gender intermittently or who openly embrace elements of both genders in their identity, are altogether excluded from *any* gender classification, and are therefore either unrecognised or recognised as 'breaking' the order of biology, and therefore as suffering from some type of pathology. Once it begins to appear that the notion of gender is in itself elusive, it becomes questionable whether transgenderism is appropriately considered as pathology, or even whether it is such a peculiar phenomenon altogether. Perhaps it is in the 'natural', obvious order of things that, once it is recognised that both sex and gender are complex occurrences, that they are interpretations of a variety of social, historical, normative, political, and biological facts, people may more and more openly recognise themselves as being *beyond birth*, more or less drastically embracing facets of different sexes and genders, permanently or intermittently. Put simply, perhaps in the past I would myself have been regarded as somehow deviant for being a breadwinner for my family and wearing 'male' clothes. Nobody now criticises me, let alone imprisons me or burns me alive (as happened to Joan of Arc), for wearing what were once male clothes, for going to work outside the house and paying for someone else to do my housework; the historical and social evolution that allows me[51] to embrace gender roles that were once thought to be the exclusive domain of men may and should now allow individuals to move across other segments of the gender continuum without much ostracism or even surprise.

4   GENDER IN CLINICAL PSYCHOLOGY AND ENDOCRINOLOGY

In clinical psychology, psychiatry, and endocrinology the notion of gender, and, more particularly, gender identity, has acquired an apparently more specific meaning.

In these contexts, gender and gender identity refer to the congruence between phenotype and the person's behaviour and feelings about oneself. Gender identity, thus, is the experience of "belonging to one sex".[52] Others define gender identity as "a person's innate sense of maleness or femaleness".[53]

In their seminal work *Man & Woman, Boy & Girl*, Money and Ehrhardt differentiate between gender identity and gender role.

> Gender Identity: The sameness, unity, and persistence of one's individuality as male, female, or ambivalent, in greater or lesser degree, especially as it is experienced in self-awareness and behaviour: gender identity is the private experience of gender role, and gender role is the public expression of gender identity.

> Gender Role: Everything that a person says and does, to indicate to others or to the self the degree that one is either male, or female, or ambivalent; it includes but is not restricted to sexual arousal and response; gender role is the public expression of gender identity, and gender identity is the private experience of gender role.[54]

In clinical psychology and endocrinology, *disorders* of gender identification refer to complex conditions in which individuals experience discomfort with their own biological sex (or what is taken to be the 'biological sex').[55] In this sense, gender dysphoria has been referred to as "sense of estrangement"[56] from one's body. Gender identity, in clinical discourses, does not typically refer to gender roles. However, clearly gender identity, even meant narrowly as the sense of congruence with our own bodies, cannot be disconnected from our acquiescence in the roles, preferences, desires, and functions that are accepted or considered as normal for men or women within a certain social and cultural context (see Chapter 3, Section 9). For this reason, some have argued that the transgender (the man trapped in a woman's body and *vice versa*) who seeks in genital reconstruction the resolution of his/her internal conflict is even more of 'a slave' of gender stereotypes than 'the mainstream' men and women.[57] I will return to this argument in Chapter 5.

Due to the fluidity of the notion of gender within various contexts, and due to the variety of models of gender development (see Chapter 3), it is difficult to reconcile different ways of understanding gender, gender identity, and disorders of gender identification. It is thus necessary to provide further clarifications relating to how gender is thought to develop and to assess the clinical implications of these various ways of thinking about gender identification.

In the next chapter, I will discuss the main theories of gender identity development. This will provide a key for understanding *atypical* gender identity development. The aim will be to understand how people may come to form a gender identity that does not conform to the expectations that others have of them. It should be noted that it is not necessarily true that so called disorders of gender identification are *biological* disorders *if gender is primarily biologically construed*. *Vice versa*, it is not necessarily true that disorders of gender identification are *not biological* disorders *if gender is primarily a social construct*. We could configure the possibility of, for example, a social construct that is rejected by an individual due to biological forces (or *vice versa*, of a biological datum that is opposed to due to social forces). However, a *dis-order* presumes the existence of *order*, and the knowledge of the *orderly* is preliminary to the understanding of the *dis-order* under analysis. Therefore, in order to understand *dis-orders* of gender development, it is necessary to understand what is an *ordered* gender development.

As we shall see further in what follows, as the binomial classification of man and woman (consequently trans *as the man trapped in a woman's body and vice versa*), also the binomial classification of *biological versus social explanations* is a misrepresentation of a more complex set of occurrences.

5   GENDER IN ARTS

I will conclude this overview of the notions of gender and gender identity with a brief account of gender in figurative arts. It is with a certain degree of humbleness that I approach the subject given that I am not an art critic. I will confine myself to illustrate and discuss the work that some artists have done,[58] especially in the 1900s, which exposes the hidden assumptions and contradictions inherent in the notion of gender, and which contributes to subverting its apparent significance or unity.

The inspiration to write this section came from the exhibition *Angels of Anarchy*, held at the Manchester City Art Gallery in 2009–2010. The title is of interest because of the thread that seems to link anarchy and transgenderism, as mentioned in the introduction to this book. *Anarchy* is a word of Greek origins. In Greek it is *anarkhia* and means *without* (an) *ruler* (arkhos). Although anarchy is typically understood as a political term, referring to those who reject the political state, its meaning may encompass all situations of absence or nonrecognition of an authority. In this wider sense, transgenderism is a form of anarchy. The other term used in the title of the exhibition, *angels*, refers to the "angelic disposition for metamorphosis", for transformation.[59] "The angelic position", writes Allmer, "is a position of in-betweenness and motion. These functions and positions are the strengths of angels: they overcome and deconstruct the paths of Western patriarchal binary thought, its hierarchical structure, replacing stability with flux, singularity with multiplicity, separation with transgression, and being with becoming and transformation".[60] Allmer, the organiser of the exhibition, wrote that the works selected were all connected by the fact that they all somewhat aimed to "overcome dualities, boundaries and binaries".[61] It is in this sense evident how these artworks are relevant to our discourse on gender and transgenders.

> Women surrealists' works explore the "intimate experience of boundaries, their construction and deconstruction"[62]. They explode and undo binary and hierarchical categorisation by "[. . .] rendering the tradition non-identical to itself",[63] perverting (in its sense of turning round) tradition, showing that tradition is not a fixed entity, but that it already inoculates its own transmutations and becomings, deconstructing itself from within, thereby producing new forms.[64]

The main aim of many of the works included in Allmer's exhibition was to contest the patriarchal society. The scope was therefore the liberation of women. The artists often chose to do so in a provocative, disturbing way: as Mary Ann Caws notes, "if it isn't sufficiently scandalous, it will absolutely change nothing about the way we see".[65]

In *Transplanted*, painted by Emmy Bridgwater in 1947, the face of the woman mixes in metamorphosis with the head of a bird. Somehow, the identity here is construed around multiplicity. Earlier, in 1927, Claude Cahun offered an interesting protest against gender stereotypes. In his *Self Portrait*,[66] for example, Cahun represents a masquerade. She plays with the notions of gender, and her works seem to aim at deconstructing gender identity, both in the subject and in the observer: we are never sure whether the subject is a male or a female, and the identity is blurred; identity is hidden under a mask, under which another identity is hidden, under which identity is not ultimately recognisable.

Many other artists across the 1900s fought against gender stereotypes and the female objectification allegedly imposed by patriarchal society. 1929's *Severed Breast from Radical Surgery in a Place Setting*, by Lee Miller, is the disquieting photograph of a real amputated breast. Miller seems to have carried the severed breast to *Vogue* magazine's studio, arranged it on a plate, and taken a shot of it. The photo has some dark irony in it, which enhances its evocative force. It clearly denounces the objectification of the female body, but it does more than this. In setting the table in a 'female fashion' (traditionally, and we would expect this to be the case in the 1920s, it is the woman who sets the table), Miller subtly and forcefully points to the implicit sacrifice and acceptance of the woman's role by the women themselves. By setting their own body as flesh for martyrdom, neatly, thus participating as actors to the whole process, women not only severe themselves, but also reinforce a social practice of subjugation and humiliation for themselves and for other women as well.[67]

In 1938 Ithell Colquhoun painted *Scylla*. Scylla, in Greek mythology, was a monster living in Sicily and threatening sailors. *Scylla* offers a poignant manipulation of genders, and it does more than this. Not only do male and female become one, but also body and landscape become each other. The painting illustrates two rocks in juxtaposition; they touch each other at the top and there is some vegetation at the bottom. The texture of the rocks, however, is actually very soft, and these two rocks come to resemble two penises that lie one on the other. Yet indeed, on another look, these two penises can also be viewed as the two thighs of a woman lying down, with flexed knees, exposing a woman's vagina. In this ingenious painting, not only do landscape and human nature amalgamate, but also male and female merge, each becoming coextensive with the other.[68]

The provocative denouncement of women's subjugation, the challenge against the rigid gender divide that nails women to unyielding gender roles, of course extends to domestic space. As we have seen earlier in this chapter, a philosophical trend suggested that by nature women are best equipped for domestic chores. The next chapter will discuss the experiments that in psychology seemed to confirm the existence of a biological substrate to gender roles. Unsurprisingly, the attack by artists against biological determinism has addressed the household as well. The house, traditionally the safe place for the woman, begins to disintegrate, and is illustrated sometimes as nightmarish, frightful, or even openly dissipating.

"Women surrealists", explains Allmer, "render unfamiliar the familiar domestic interiors associated [. . .] with the ideologically seen 'natural' environments of women. [. . .] The everyday domestic interior is emptied out and returns as a space full of haunting and nightmarish potentials—potentials for transformation and becoming".[69]

In 1943 Dorothea Tanning painted *Eine Kleine Nachtmusik*.[70] This painting represents a familiar environment, probably a hotel, but one that is oppressive and fearful. In this work, she portrays two young girls haunted by the threatening atmosphere of the place. The two girls seem to fight with a giant sunflower (symbol of surrealism, after André Bréton published the poem *Sunflower*),[71] declaring that women can define and reinvent themselves against every tradition or movement and categorisation.[72] Here the meaning is not only artistic: it represents an outcry over authority, with its sexual, social, and political meanings.

The notion of female identity recurs across the 1900s works. Kay Sage, in 1955, painted *Tomorrow Is Never*. In a space that is surreal, but frightful and empty, the female form is wrapped in a veil, silenced and exposed at the same time, and trapped in structures that resemble skyscrapers but also cages. This seems to express the nonfixity of female identity, in spite of the imprisonment in the domestic space suffered by women, and from which, it seems in the painting, there is little hope for evasion.

Later in the century, the photographer Francesca Woodman offered a poignant and striking continuation of the deconstruction of domestic space. *House 3*, a photo dated 1976, represents the domestic space, the 'women's space' as disintegrated or *disintegrating*. The photo illustrates a bare room, blown up and with scratched walls and floors, and the figure of a woman that is distinguishable but not clearly visible, as she is evaporating in the rotten house environment. Not only is the space decadent, which seems to illustrate how the dogma of the blessed family home is shattered, but the woman herself is volatilised in it.[73] In a later photograph, dated 1977–1978, Woodman offers a perhaps more complex picture of domestic life. Here a female figure hangs on the ledge of a door frame; her face is not visible. She has the lightness of an ascending angel and the brutality of a female body crucified in the house. A discarded cloth suggests a rejection of traditional domestic labour, implying the 'choice' of being crucified, the drastic decision of renouncing identity altogether for the sake of rejection of an assigned identity.[74]

Many other artists have offered interesting ideas for thinking about gender, gender identity, gender roles, and the relationship between the individual as gendered, by reason of biological attributes, and the engendering society. I haven't done justice of course to all artists who contributed to challenging the gender boundaries. This brief account is meant to offer some additional insight into the meanings of gender and widen further the survey of various presentations of gender in different contexts. Hopefully this overview, albeit brief and necessarily incomplete, can broaden the perspective from which the notion of gender, with its boundaries and its meaning, may be considered.

It may be objected that the artworks challenging genders say little about transgenderism, as they refer mainly to *women's versus men's roles*. However, these works are important and relevant to our context because, by deconstructing the notion of female gender, inevitably they question the notion of gender altogether: its fixity; immutability; the normative values that it acquires; the meanings that it has for the 'genderised' individual; and thus the psychological, moral, social, and political significance that *any* notion of gender inevitably has.

By looking closely at how the notions of gender and gender identity are used, it has been possible to discover the vagueness of the notions themselves. This vagueness is not a problem to be overcome, but a fact to be recognised and valued: gender and gender identity have polyvalent meanings; they reflect the many different ways in which each individual may develop. There is not one meaning attached to gender or one 'normal' way of developing as a man or a woman. Being a man or a woman has a diverse meaning for different people, and has a diverse meaning at different stages of one's life.

6   CONCLUSIONS

I will desert your armies. I will freely circulate in the intermediate space. We'll see if your gods or your bullets can drive me out of it.

(Claude Cahun, 1930)[75]

Gender is a vague notion, inherently indeterminate and *intermediate*. It refers to the substance of beings; to the masculine, feminine, or neutral classes of nouns; to the category of belonging of human beings; to social roles; to expectations; to the relationship between what one feels one is and to some biological facts (such as one's chromosomal and genetic makeup). I have illustrated in this chapter the complexities relating to this notion and to the notion of gender identity. There is not a univocal answer to what gender identity is. It does not surprise us, therefore, that there may be confusion on what transgenderism or a dis-order of gender identity may be. Does it have to do with biology? Is it caused by misguided social, or perhaps parental, cues? What is the 'order' on which this 'dis-order' can be tested?

Sociological and gender studies, with their philosophical backgrounds, have provided important clues to begin to understand the complexities inherent to the notions of gender and gender identity. Appreciation of such complexity is necessary in order to disentangle, later in the book, the issues related to gender identification, both typical and atypical.

These various studies, in spite of their sometimes important differences, have in fact one point in common: they have all pointed out that, whether or not the notions of 'man' and 'woman' are grounded in biology (in essential or biological differences between human males and human females, rather than in social constructs), gender roles, the places that people occupy in society, their rights and worth are also, to a significant extent, a matter of social interpretation.

An overview of these studies, thus, challenges us to reconsider the very meaning of the notions of 'man' and 'woman'. The debates on the notion of gender highlight the very fact that the binomial classic distinction between male and female genders is amendable and subject to criticism and rational scrutiny. This could be true even if some differences between human males and females can be grounded in biology. This recasting of sex and gender as dynamic, subject to historical and cultural interpretations, has important normative implications: pointing at the social construction of gender means that people are not ill or disordered if they embrace different segments of various genders in their identity. The fuller implications of this will be examined throughout the book.

There are many more elements of gender development and of atypical gender identification that need to be explored and understood. In the next chapter, I will discuss the main theories of gender development and the clinical and normative repercussions that these theories may have.

3 Gender Identity Development

At dawn will be magic, will be miraculous breasts.

(F. De André, 'Princesa', 1996)[1]

1 INTRODUCTION

The song 'Princesa' is inspired by the real story of Fernanda Farias, who called herself *Princesa, Princess*. [2] The song narrates Fernanda's story, born in Latin America as Fernando, and of the *chiaroscuro* (*light and shade*) in which she grew up, which evokes not only the objective condition of street children, who find respite from the heat of the Latin summers in the shades of the tree branches, but metaphorically illustrates the ambiguity of her own perception of her gender identity as a child. In the song, his mother realises that Fernandino behaves like a girl, but she does not worry. It will be *instinct or life* to remind him that he was born as a boy. But in the face of the mother's hopes, Fernando as a child continues to dream about being a girl. Fernanda will later emigrate clandestinely to Italy, to "correct her fate", that is, to have medical treatment and "a body that looks like her". She will work as a prostitute and will end up in prison. After her release, in 1999, Princesa sadly committed suicide.

Before analysing in greater details the situation of children with atypical gender (Chapter 4), in this chapter I will discuss how gender identity is thought to develop. Fernanda illustrates a case of atypical gender identification in childhood which persists in adulthood. Fernanda knows right from her childhood that she has a predominant feminine side that other boys either do not have or do not recognise. But how does the process of gender identification occur in 'normal' circumstances? Answering this question is preliminary to the understanding of what happens to people who 'depart' from what is regarded as 'normal' development.

In this chapter I provide an account of the main explanations of gender identity development. Each of them, as we shall see, captures some important elements of gender identity development. However, none of them should be accepted *bona fide* and used with unreserved reverence to direct clinical practice. We will see that adopting *tout court* a theory of gender identity development in clinical practice may be risky. Blind acceptance of one theoretical model can be, and has been proven to be, potentially harmful. It is therefore imperative that a degree of scepticism grounds clinical approaches to gender variance.

I will conclude this chapter by showing that there is no unequivocal answer to how gender identity develops. Gender identity is one of the aspects of personal identity. Gender identity is the result of a complex interplay of various factors: social, biological, and perhaps of other natures as well (historical, cultural, cognitive, and so on). The perception of our own gender (like the perception of other elements of ourselves) may also depend on various personal elements, including cognitive responses (*who one thinks one is*), affective responses (*who one feels one is*), and volitional responses (*who one wants to be*).[3] All these factors combine themselves in a unique way in each individual to create the person that each feels and thinks one is and wants to be. In this sense, being a part of a gender minority is as uncomplicated (or as complicated) as being a 'straight' woman or man. All the processes of gender development are equally complex (or simple), equally unique, and equally legitimate.

2   THEORIES OF GENDER DEVELOPMENT

The process by which children learn their gender identity is known as *sex typing*. There is an agreement on the fact that a gender identity is stable and constant by the age of six or seven.[4] It has been suggested that children as young as two years of age already possess substantive knowledge of sex stereotypes, and that such knowledge is highly correlated with the understanding of their own gender identity.[5] Indeed even during infancy, boys and girls often show marked preferences for stereotypical male or female toys.[6]

How gender develops is much more controversial: is gender somehow written in our genes and chromosomes? How significant is the contribution of biology and that of society?

There are, broadly speaking, three models of gender development:

1. the biological model
2. the social model
3. the biosocial model

This list is not meant to cover all theories of gender development, but there are significant elements in various theories that allow these to be grouped under these three general headings. At the end of this chapter I will also provide a synthetic account of the sociobiological theory, Freud's psychoanalytic theory, and the cognitive-developmental theory (CDT), and I will discuss briefly cultural relativism.[7] I focus on the social, biological, and biosocial model, as these models help us to understand the following points, which are the central concerns of our analysis:

1. Whether the process of sex typing is scientifically clear.
2. Whether gender derives from *nature or nurture*, and what the relative contribution of each eventually is.
3. Whether this tells us anything about transgenderism.

4. Whether this tells us anything normatively or clinically: more clearly, if biology explained transgenderism, would this mean that medical treatment (for example, hormonal or surgical treatments) is clinically and ethically justified (or morally required)? *Vice versa*, if transgenderism is a social construct, would this mean that medical interventions are unethical and should be replaced by social interventions?

In order to answer these questions, and, indeed, in order to articulate them more precisely before beginning to answer them, it is important to understand how sex typing and gender identity are thought to occur.

As just mentioned, I group together theories that share fundamental points: for example, the social model incorporates constructionism,[8] deconstructionism,[9] the theory of the sexual difference, and post-modern feminism.[10] The works of very different authors are subsumed under this model. I group under the social model all the theories whose core idea is that *the main determinant* of gender identity formation is the social/familial input, rather than biology. I do the same with the other models: I group together different theories that share a fundamental core idea.

This broad overview of theories of gender development will equip us to understand the grounds that have historically been used to frame clinical interventions for transgenderism.

3 THE BIOLOGICAL MODEL

The main assumption of the biological model is that *gender identity* is mainly determined by biological forces.

The theoretical background to this approach is to be found in various philosophical and sociological theories, in particular from the 1700s onwards (see Chapter 2). August Comte, for example, the father of modern sociology, proposed a theory of society based on the natural makeup of men and women. He wrote:

> The social function of women becomes [. . .] a necessary consequence of their very nature. The positive regime [the social regime that Comte hoped to realise] assigns to women a noble social function, which is both public and private at the same time. Without leaving the family they must, in their own way, participate in the moderating power with philosophers and proletariat, giving up, more than they have to, every directional power, including the domestic one.[11]
> The fundamental role assigned to the woman is [. . .] a vast systematic development of her particular nature [. . .] The natural law that assigns to the affective sex [women] an existence that is essentially domestic has never been gravely altered. This law is so real that it has always spontaneously prevailed.[12]

Comte believed that nature shapes social roles, and therefore society as a whole. Of course, if nature determines the role of the woman, this implies at least two things:

1. That nature determines the role of men as well.
2. That those who do not recognise themselves in this classification are *against nature*, and therefore deviant, wrong, or ill.

Comte is thought to be the predecessor of so called *functionalism*. According to functionalism, society is an organism comparable to the human body. In society various elements contribute to general harmony, in the same way as it happens within the human body. In this theoretical framework the echo of biological sciences is very notable. At the time in which biological sciences acquired standing (particularly during the nineteenth and twentieth centuries) many intellectuals drew parallels between the physical body and the social body. Amongst those are Herbert Spencer (1820–1903), Vilfredo Pareto (1848–1923), Emile Durkheim (1858–1917), and Talcott Parsons (1902–1979). The common denominator amongst them is that they all believed that biological and sexual differences exist between men and women, and that these correspond to differences in attitudes, preferences, and abilities. This explains why women and men have different skills and succeed in different activities, which are functional to the order, cohesion, and harmony of society.

Various clinical studies seem to have given strength to these theoretical frameworks. John Bowlby,[13] for example, argued that some differences in the attitudes and behaviours of males and females are genetically transmitted instincts. At least some of the roles linked to gender are, according to Bowlby, instinctual and biological and not socially determined. On this line, Simon Baron-Cohen wrote: "The female brain is predominantly 'hard-wired' for empathy. The male brain is predominantly 'hard- wired' for understanding and building systems".[14] Gender role is innate and biologically determined, according to the biological model. The preference for different toys and activities, observed in very young girls and boys, is an indication of this. The differences are also physical: male babies are generally bigger; boys often sleep less and cry more, and are generally more active, whereas girls start talking earlier than boys and so on.

Several studies have explored the psychological attributes belonging to each sex and children's sex differences.[15] Richard Green has provided a review of these studies. Some of these illustrate that already at the age of ten to eighteen months, boys tend to identify themselves with boys and girls with girls. For example, in one study babies of this age were presented with some pictures of faces of infants of the same sex and of the other sex. It was observed that boys looked at boys' faces longer and girls looked at girls' faces longer. This was regarded as an indication that, even at this early stage, babies have some recognition of "like me" and "not like me".[16] It also appears that boys and girls begin to prefer 'sex-typed' toys by the age of one year, and that, around the age of three and a half and four and a half, boys prefer to play with boys and girls with girls.[17]

According to some studies, these differences are mainly biological. Research on animals (for example, on birdsongs, on urinary posture in canines, even in fish and in mammalians such as rhesus monkeys) suggests that sexually dimorphic behaviour has a strong relationship with brain structure and hormones, including prenatal exposure to hormones.[18]

Zucker notes that prenatal exposure to androgens "plays a role in the pattern of masculinisation that has been observed across a variety of behavioural domains".[19] Experimental evidence from animal studies suggests that altering the balance of various hormones changes the gender role behaviour. The behavioural systems that appear affected include nurturing ('maternalism'), affiliation (nonsexual peer relations), aggression, and activity levels, all of which show normative sex differences and which, at least in lower animals, have been shown to be affected by experimental manipulations in exposure to prenatal sex hormones, including androgens.

Thus, according to the biological paradigm, gender development is primarily determined by the person's biological makeup. Sex differences (see Chapter 2) determine children's preferences for toys, activities, even clothes, and determine subsequent preferences for roles within the family and in society (work, parenting, caring, and nurturing activities versus financially oriented occupations or competitive pursuits).[20] The biological model is also called *essentialist*, in that it assumes that *in their very essence* people differ due to biological forces. One implication of this is that rearing cannot modify biologically determined behaviours and attitudes. Another implication is that where gender differentiation does not occur as expected, it is possible that some biological alteration may have occurred, for example, in hormonal exposure during foetal life.

KEY POINTS: THE BIOLOGICAL (OR ESSENTIALIST) MODEL

- Biological/sexual differences exist between men and women.
- These correspond to differences in attitudes, preferences, and abilities.
- From the 1700s onward various philosophers engaged with discourses on the 'natural' differences between men and women.
- Bowlby: some differences and gendered behaviours in males and females are genetically transmitted instincts.
- Children's preferences for toys and activities indicate sex difference.
- Physical differences indicate and are a prelude to gender differences.
- Rearing cannot modify biologically determined behaviours/attitudes.
- Maternalism, aggression, and other gender related behaviours are modified in other animals by manipulations of exposure to prenatal hormones.

4   THE SOCIAL MODEL

Diametrically opposed to the biological model is the social model. As anticipated before, there are various explanations of gender identity development that appeal to the influence of society. I will group them all together
in spite of their differences, as what matters here is their core idea: the main
hypothesis of social models of gender development is that both gender role
and gender identity are mainly *social constructs*. For this reason, social
models of gender are also called *constructionist* models (sometimes they
are called *deconstructionist*, although constructionism and deconstructionism are slightly different theories. See notes 7 and 8). Against essentialist models, these argue that gender roles are not *a datum*, an inner state
relating to one's biology, but conventions.

Scott, for example, argued that the categories of men and women are
meaningless. They are ideal notions, which are filled in with mental representations that effectively deny people the possibility to be who they
really are.[21]

The social model has, of course, been embraced by many feminists,
whose work has been aimed at dismantling the idea that the traditional
roles assigned to women, and the subjugation of women, can be justified on
grounds of their physical differences.

There is an important distinction to make here: according to some
authors, such as, for example, Luce Irigaray, there are indeed gender differences and these are effectively based on our biological makeup: women
are incontrovertibly weaker than men on average, they gestate children,
produce milk to feed them, and so on. This explains at least some of the
different roles that men and women tend to acquire in society. However,
Irigaray insists that these differences should be valued and dignified, rather
than used to subjugate women. Moreover, importantly, Irigaray is careful
to talk of *at least two sexes*. Thus Irigaray recognises the possibility of,
potentially, pluralities of unrecognised gender identities.[22]

According to pure constructionists, such as, for example, Judith Butler,[23]
gender is a *mere construct*. The conceptual difference here is important, as
important as the practical consequences of this are. For those who believe
that there is such a thing as a gender difference (such as Irigaray), a just
society is one that acknowledges such differences and even codifies it (for
example, with the recognition of *sexed or gendered rights*). Men and
women cannot be treated *equally* because they are substantially different.
For the pure constructionists, instead, a just society is one that transcends
sex or gender differences entirely, and that allows for the proliferation of a
variety of sex and gender identities, where laws and social policies are *gender neutral*. As Feinberg suggests: "Sex categories should be removed from
all basic identification papers—from driver's licences to passports—and
because the right of each person to define their own sex is so basic, it should
be eliminated from birth certificates as well".[24] The social expectations

relating to gender are so strong and deeply embodied in Western societies that the possibility of a newborn baby who is neither male nor female is still legally difficult to reconcile. This inability of many legal systems to forecast the possibility of accommodating children of unknown gender often determines the fate of those who are born with ambiguous genitalia. As we shall see later in this chapter, clinical practice often favours the elimination of ambiguity at birth. Babies born with ambiguous genitalia often receive 'corrective' surgery and hormonal treatment, which enables the parents to register the child as a boy or a girl and raise him/her according to social genderised precepts. "For questions of inheritance, legitimacy, paternity, succession to title, and eligibility for certain professions to be determined, modern Anglo-Saxon legal systems require that newborns be registered as either male or female".[25]

In spite of these important differences, theories within the social model share the core idea that society determines gender roles and identities *how we know them*. What it is to be a woman and a man, now and here, is primarily based on social precepts and sanctions. Whereas it seems incontrovertible that there are behaviours and attitudes that are more often seen in men/boys and others more often seen in women/girls, these are primarily socially construed. Margaret Mead, for example, noted that the degree of aggression in men varies across different socio-cultural settings, and that the degree of gentleness and nurturance expected of women fluctuates across different societies.[26] Thus, whether or not biology determines some traits, like aggression, these are always filtered, reinforced, or inhibited by social and cultural variables.

The *queer* theory (*queer* is a word of German origins, which literally means *transversal, oblique, diagonal*)[27] insists on the same point. The queer theory borrows from Michel Foucault[28] the idea that identities that are sometimes presented as *natural* are complex socio-cultural establishments. Hence queer studies are interested in all phenomena of hybrid gender formation, in new bodily latitudes and marginalities (cross dressers, hermaphrodites, androgynous bodies, and so on).

Gender, thus, is a social construct (whether or not some 'structural' or behavioural differences exist that can be grounded in biology), and gender identity is not determined primarily by the biological facts, but by the social reinforcements of behaviours, attitudes, and preferences, which are constructed as precepts for birth sex. Gender identities are to a major extent created by others: by the parents at a developmental stage; by educators at a schooling stage; by the interaction with peers; and, more generally, by the social responses to the sex appearance of a baby.

Children learn the behaviour that their society, in many understated and implicit ways, expects of people of their sex. Lorber showed how parents model gender behaviour, encourage children to behave appropriately, and reinforce them when they do.[29] At birth one of the first preoccupations of many parents is determination of sex: as soon as sex is assigned, children are treated differently according to their sex. The child, in turn, responds with feelings and behaviours that are congruent to these triggers.[30] Adults, often without realising it, behave in a different way with the same baby depending on whether they think the baby is male or female. For example, in a study discussed by Green, fathers, observed while interacting with twelve-month-old boys, were more likely to offer them trucks rather than dolls, whereas girls were given equally trucks and dolls.[31] From the time that parents learn whether the new baby is a boy or girl, many aspects of the way it is treated will be influenced by its sex.[32]

CASE HISTORY 1: BETH AND ADAM[33]

Will et al. observed a group of young women interacting with a girl, Beth, aged five months. Women were seen smiling often to the child and offering her dolls to play. The girl was said to be 'sweet'. They then observed five different young mothers with a baby called Adam, aged five months. The mothers were offering Adam trains and showed reactions that were remarkably different to those of the previous group. Beth and Adam were of course the same baby, dressed differently.[34] Thus children are motivated to talk in the way that is prescribed by their gender and to adopt the mannerisms believed to be appropriate to the birth sex by their social groups.[35]

Bandura performed a number of clinical studies on gender identity development. He observed that gender identity development is heavily based on external sanctions: parents in many cultures provide play experiences that are sex typed. Bandura coined the term *social learning theory*. According to him, children learn to behave differently if they are boys and girls *because they are treated differently*. Children monitor their behaviour against the expected standards and feel pride in performing gender role consistent behaviour, even if there is no explicit external sanction or praise.[36]

A number of studies suggest that gender roles are internalised by very young children, and that the environmental (implicit or explicit) sanctions shape the children's response.[37] Bussey and Bandura, for example, studied three- and four-year-old nursery children. They asked the children to evaluate gender typed behaviour of peers (from videotapes) playing with 'masculine' or 'feminine' toys. Even younger children showed disapproval of gender inconsistent behaviour (for example, boys playing with dolls).[38] Lloyd and Duveen studied 120 children aged eighteen months to three years old and arrived at similar conclusions.[39]

The social model, as we shall see in the next section, has had an important impact on clinical practice.

KEY POINTS: THE SOCIAL MODEL

- Gender role and gender identity are *social constructs*.
- Scott: The categories of men and women are ideal notions.
- Irigaray: sex differences do exist but should be valued and dignified, rather than used to subjugate women.
- Butler: sex differences are pure constructions.
- Bandura: gender development is heavily based on external sanctions (social learning theory). Children monitor their behaviour against the expected standards and feel pride in performing gender role consistent behaviour, even in the absence of open sanction or praise.
- Gender roles are internalised by very young children.

4.1   The Social Model and Clinical Practice

The idea that gender identity is not innate and can be moulded by upbringing has had significant impact upon clinical practice. Studies such as those reported in Section 4 have guided for a few decades the treatment of children born with ambiguous genitalia, at least in the US (for a description of these conditions, called Disorders of Sex Development [DSDs], see Chapter 2).

Money, [40] for example, treated a number of intersex children on the basis of the idea that if gender is reassigned within a critical period (normally two and a half to three years of age) the child will suffer no psychological harm (children whose gender is assigned later were thought to be less likely to adjust without complications). Insofar as parents also believe in the gender of rearing, a child raised in a certain gender will typically conform to that gender. Regardless of the chromosomal heritage, gender will develop without ambiguity in the gender of rearing.[41] Gender is mainly a matter of nurture and not nature. Clinical literature reports cases of people who are chromosomal males, with external phenotype as females, who are raised according to genital appearance and who identify unequivocally with the gender of rearing.[42]

Zucker writes: "in a study of 105 hermaphrodites, Money et al. (1957) found that only 5 of 105 patients had a 'gender role and orientation [that] was ambiguous and deviant from the sex of assignment and rearing' (p.333). Thus, Money et al. concluded that 'the sex of assignment and rearing is consistently and conspicuously a more reliable prognosticator of a hermaphrodite's gender role and orientation than is the chromosomal sex, the gonadal sex, the hormonal sex, the accessory internal reproductive morphology, or the ambiguous morphology of the external genitalia' (p.333)."[43]

However, some unsuccessful clinical cases have challenged not only the practice of early surgical treatment for intersex, but also the validity of the social model, especially as a basis for clinical practice.[44]

The sad case of John/Joan is famous.[45]

CASE HISTORY 2: JOHN/JOAN

During a circumcision operation carried out at eight months on two twins, the penis of one of the boys was severed. Money, the surgeon, advised on reconstructing a vagina and raising the child as a girl. The boy was never happy being 'a girl'. He later took the name of David Reimer and had reassignment surgery to male. David accused Money of having condemned him to a childhood of humiliation and misery. David wrote: "The organ that appears to be critical to psychosexual development and adaptation is not the genitalia but the brain".[46] David committed suicide in 2004.

Analyses of this and other similar cases indicate that gender identity cannot in all cases be moulded by upbringing.

4.2   What Lessons Can Be Drawn?

The studies examined in the preceding bring to light the complexities inherent to gender identity development. This suggests one important thing: the theoretical approaches discussed here may capture some elements of the complex process of gender identification, but should not be used with absolute deference in clinical practice. A rigid application of a theoretical model can have severely negative consequences for the person's well-being. A significant degree of scepticism should drive clinical practice. Nobody knows exactly how gender identity should be understood and how it develops, and, therefore, paying a blind tribute to one theoretical model can have potentially hideous consequences.

With regard to the clinical approach to children with DSDs, the Intersex Society of North America suggests that any medical intervention should occur when the child's gender can be predicted, and when the child is mature enough to make an informed decision.[47] DSDs are only in a minority of cases associated with health risks, and therefore the mutilation of the body of the baby is not justified by medical necessity, and is, therefore, at least morally dubious. Of course, social ostracism and parental inability to cope with the situation are factors that may be taken into account when considering what is in the best interests of a child.[48] However, the blind application of the social model to clinical practice can, on evidence, no longer be justified.

Whereas these considerations concern DSDs and not children with atypical gender directly, they are relevant to their case as well: the social model may capture important aspects of gender identity development but it is not sufficient, on its own, to explain it. It would, therefore, be inappropriate to conclude, simply based on this model, that gender variance is purely or primarily a product of social or parental triggers. The clinical implications of this are clear: if gender variance was primarily the result of social forces, then it could be possible in principle to amend gender dysphoria and 'correct' it without necessarily intervening on the person's body. Perhaps 'corrective' interventions *should* be aimed primarily at amending the social forces responsible for the 'deviation'. Instead, as we have seen earlier in this book, gender identity development encompasses much more than social forces, without denying that those social factors that are responsible for people's suffering ought to be amended. I will further suggest that transgenderism is not *per se* a bad outcome, and not necessarily one to be 'corrected', if by 'corrected' one means to bring the person back to identify him/herself with the gender assigned at birth. I shall return to this point later in the book. Let us, for now, continue the examination of the models of gender development.

5   THE BIOSOCIAL MODEL

In a detailed review of animal studies and studies of gender identification of people with various forms of DSDs, Zucker found that women with congenital androgen hyperplasia (CAH; see Chapter 2) have less satisfaction with their gender than control groups, regardless of upbringing. This seems to support the hypothesis of a significant biological contribution to gender formation. But Zucker also notes that studies on rats show that "the average number of neurons in the corpus callosum of rats shows a significant sex difference. However, this typical sex difference is exquisitely sensitive to, and modified by, the rearing environment".[49] Zucker thus reaches an important conclusion: the development of gender encompasses both biological forces and social norms. Archer and Lloyds, similarly, write:

> Development is a complex process that must ultimately involve the interplay of both [biological and social forces]. But, for the purposes of identifying specific influences that really make a difference, researchers have tended to forget this wider picture. For example, the social learning tradition involves concentrating on the process of imitation and ignoring the impact of prenatal androgens because these are regarded as unimportant in explaining what is imitated and under what circumstances. Biological approaches concentrating on the influence of prenatal androgens would tend to ignore details of the social environment, since these are regarded as unimportant compared with the hormonal influence. What is implicit in both research strategies is a belief that the variable under investigation is the main controlling influence on the behavioural outcome being investigated.[50]

However, we have seen in the preceding that the 'split' between models is somehow sharp and that the implications for clinical practice can also be significant. Thus, it is crucial to bear in mind that both models contribute to our understanding of gender identity development and cannot be taken in isolation. None of these models should be applied with absolute deference to clinical practice.

Gender development is a complex process that is the result, variable and dynamic (open to changes over time), of an interplay involving both biological and social factors, as well as individual interpretations, preferences, wishes, and needs. Gender identity is a part of a broader notion of identity, which is formed in a unique way based probably on biology, on social interactions, and on the original manner in which each individual makes sense of what it is to be him/herself within the context in which s/he lives.

The notion of 'identity', like the notion of 'gender', has been widely debated both in psychology and philosophy. In psychology, the notion of identity is generally used in concomitance with 'self-concept'. Several studies have provided various accounts of when and how people, as well as animals, acquire a sense of 'who they are'. Researchers have studied the cognitive structures that allow self-reflection and organisation of information about oneself.[51] Studies on animals and children have attempted to disentangle the way in which, and the phases of life at which, individuals form a concept of their own identity (who they are, how they are differentiated from others, and what responses they can elicit in others and in the surrounding environment). Identity, in broad terms, is thought to comprise self-image, social roles, personality traits, self-esteem, autobiographical memory, age, *and gender.*

Gender is thus one of the many elements of 'who one is', and wedges in the concept of self with various other facts and interpretations. Gender includes activities and interests, relationships, verbal and nonverbal communication styles, and values.[52] Gender, thus, cannot be regarded as a stable concept. Both the concept of gender and how people identify and express themselves change over time and according to social and cultural values and norms. Males and females thus are not, and cannot be, homogeneous groups. As each individual is unique and different to any other, his or her way of being 'a male' or 'a female' will necessarily be unique and different.[53]

However, gender cannot always be moulded by rearing, because the biological facts are also determinant.

KEY POINTS: BIOSOCIAL MODEL

- Sex and gender result from an interaction of biological and social forces.
- The relative contribution is not assessable.
- Because the social contribution is important, gender is relative to the socio-cultural context.

5.1 Biosocial Models and Clinical Practice

If gender identity is a process, which each individual develops according to a complex interplay of subjective features and preferences, biology, and social forces, it follows that gender variance is not a purely intra-psychic phenomenon or a condition that has to do purely with something that happens within the individual (dodgy chromosomes or genes, dysfunctional upbringing, imbalances in prenatal hormones), but is a relational condition, that is, a condition that depends on the rapport of the individual with his or her familial/social context. *Who one is* is neither purely caused by biology nor solely socially constructed: clearly, *who one is* results from biological and social factors and from the unique way in which each individual processes, interprets, internalises, and expresses those factors. Gender variances are *ways of being*, and thus   position themselves along a continuum of legitimate expressions of *who one is*.[54]

It follows that variations in gender identification are as normal or as deviant as it is to be unequivocally woman or man. All processes of gender identification are equally complicated (and equally simple). They all require a complex and long process of negotiation between preferences, inclinations, biological makeup, social expectations, personal experiences, and acquisition of social roles.

Not coincidentally, a large part of the suffering of people with transgenderism and in those born with various forms of intersex (and also in those who care for them) is related to the often understated assumptions about how each of us is expected to be, namely, a man or a woman with adoption of roles that are congruent with the biological sex (see Chapter 5). The very notion of 'transgender' or 'transsexual' may contain the germs of a profound misunderstanding, in that it is often understood as the condition of being 'trapped in the wrong body', as if switching to the other pole may resolve the predicaments. Gender variance encompasses instead various forms and ways of being, "multiple social identities", [55] as Bolin puts it (see Chapter 2).

Before concluding this chapter, I will give a brief account of four other theories of gender identity development, which have been influential in clinical practice: the sociobiological theory, Freud's psychoanalytic theory, CDT, and gender-schematic processing theory (GSPT).[56]

6 FREUD'S PSYCHOANALYTIC APPROACH

Freud's theory of gender development is a part of his theory of psychosexual development. According to Freud, sex and gender identity becomes stable with the resolution of the Oedipus complex (for boys) and of the Electra complex[57] (for girls). Freud borrows the names of Oedipus and Electra from the Greek mythology. In the tragedy *Oedipus the King*,

Sophocles narrates how Oedipus kills his father Laius (not knowing he is his son), and marries his mother, Jocasta. According to Freud, both boys and girls form a strong attachment to their mother, who is their first love object. At around the age of three, boys do not want to share their mother with anyone and become jealous and competitive against their father. However, boys are aware that their fathers are bigger and stronger than they are, and they form an unconscious fear of castration, a fear that their father will eventually cut off their penis. The boy resolves this fear by repressing his desire for the mother and identifying with the father. This identification with the most powerful, with the potential aggressor, coincides with adoption of gendered (male) behaviours. The girl, instead, begins her process of gender formation with the unconscious belief that she has already been castrated and holds the mother responsible for it. This process leads to what Freud called *penis envy*. When the girl realises that her wish for a penis is unrealistic, she substitutes it with the wish for a baby. She thus starts loving the father and identifying herself with the mother, in the hope that the father will give her a baby. The resolution of these conflicts leads the child to identify him/herself with the same sex parent. At this point, the child acquires a superego and a stable sex and gender identity. If this process is inhibited by traumatic experiences, sex and gender identification are likely to be inhibited. Therefore, where people show problems in sex and gender identification, according to Freud's theory, it is highly likely that the Oedipus and Electra complexes have not been resolved appropriately.[58]

Although Freud's theory has inspired many to explore human behaviour from a novel perspective, the Freudian theory of sex and gender development has been largely criticised (see also Chapter 5 for more on psychoanalytic and psychodynamic therapies of gender dysphoria). Golombok, in particular, noticed that gender identification occurs in children much earlier than the stage at which Freud postulated the resolution of the Oedipus complex to occur. More importantly, children raised in atypical families, in fatherless settings, for example, or brought up by gay or lesbian couples, have a sex and gender identification that is comparable to those raised by one woman and one man.[59] This seems to discredit the idea that the resolution of the Oedipus and Electra complexes, as imagined by Freud, produces a stable sex and gender orientation, as these children raised in atypical families obviously cannot resolve the presumed complexes in the way described by Freud, and, according to his theory, presumably all of them should suffer from some disorder of gender identification.

Despite the fact that Freud's interpretation of gender development has had limited success, the (perhaps more raw) idea that transgenderism results from situations of family conflicts that the child articulates through rejection of their gender of assignment has instead had more fortune, [60] and perhaps responds to an ordinary unrefined intuition, that if children have these 'problems', they must have encountered some hardship in upbringing.

Although this idea may be a part of ordinary discourse, there is no evidence that upbringing causes transgenderism.

It is also important to note that, within the psychoanalytic framework, *successful* therapy is the one that brings the person back within the binary *male or female* polarity. For example, Haber reports the case of a three-year-and-nine-month-old boy who wished to become a girl. He was brought to psychoanalytic therapy, which lasted five years. Haber reports:

> Developmental arrest seemed to occur during the anal rapprochement and oedipal phases that led to observable cross gender strivings by two and half years of age. The [. . .] mother's childhood wish for a sister, the mother's adult wish for a daughter, a shared fantasy between mother and child, identification with the perceived power and beauty of mother and grandmother [. . .] interwoven in the background was the impact of an emotionally absent father, a dying grandfather, and an accident-prone uncle. This paternal matrix seemed to discourage budding masculinity and encourage feminine identification [. . .] The gradual resolution of the conflicted wish to be a girl was supplanted by the emergence of *appropriate* gender identification. A two-year follow up appeared to confirm [. . .] consolidation of *stable* gender development.[61]

Here the assumption is that, structurally, the development of gender, when appropriate, will lead a child to mature into a man or into a woman, in a stable way across time, depending on the biological sex, provided that the family is functional enough to promote *adequate* adjustment. If the process (perhaps in the presence of an accident-prone uncle!) has a different outcome, then gender identification is *inappropriate*. The binary distinction here is strong and rigid, with an implicit precept that only two genders are functional to human well-being, and that only one 'healthy' way of developing exists: the one that is in line with the biological sex and that is stable across one person's life. If the outcome of therapy is stability of gender identification, in congruence with the biological sex, then therapy is *successful*. Instability of gender, gender rebellion, gender nomadism, gender transition, and ambiguity are *family and clinical failures*.

The model does not account for the fact that biological sex itself is not straightforward (see Chapter 2). Moreover, this theory does not consider that transgenderism occurs in many functional families where only one child, and not all, is transgender. Finally, within this approach gender variance is considered as pathological, at the best as a functional adaptation to a dysfunctional setting. This approach therefore is flawed, in that it assumes what needs to be demonstrated (that transgenderism is indeed pathology) and risks basing clinical practice on this (inherently discriminatory and unsubstantiated) assumption.

7   COGNITIVE-DEVELOPMENTAL THEORY (CDT): KOHLBERG

Kohlberg's theory suggests that gender, as well as sex attitudes, are not determined by biology or socio-cultural norms, but by the way the child organises his or her own social world. The determinant factor is therefore the cognitive organisation of each individual child. In this sense, CDT should be placed within the biosocial model. It allows for the significance of both external sanctions and reinforcements and biological facts, but it also stresses the importance of how each of us, as unique individuals, articulate, model, and experience the biological facts and environmental cues. Children, in other words, *discover* what *makes* them boys or girls.

Gender identification occurs, according to Kohlberg, in various stages:

- *Gender labelling*: around the age of two to three and a half years, children become aware of their own sex, but believe that this can change.
- *Gender stability*: around the age of three and a half to four and a half years children begin to form awareness of the fact that gender does not change. However, most children at this stage rely on superficial signs (such as hair length) and therefore may get easily confused in identifying people's gender.
- *Gender consistency*: between four and a half and seven years of age children gain full awareness of gender stability. They will know that sex remains the same.[62]

Kohlberg also added an important hypothesis: once a child has reached the stage of gender consistency, s/he will *value* behaviours and characteristics associated with his or her own gender. At this stage children identify themselves with adult figures of the same sex and want to adopt those features that appear associated with their gender identity. This is how gender identity is formed and crystallised.

Later studies confirmed the importance of cognitive factors in the development of gender identity.[63] Inspired by Kohlberg and Bem, Martin and Halverson[64] refined a Gender Schema Theory (GST). According to this theory, the emergence of gender stereotypes in children is a normal consequence of children's information processing. The 'schema' is the mental structure that guides the processing of information and experience. Children construct schemas that are 'in group' (same sex) and 'out group' (opposite sex). These groups include broad categorisations of activities, behaviours, and clothes, which they attribute to being a boy or a girl. The less complex the schema, the more rigid the stereotype. Therefore, younger children often have more rigid classifications and gender distinctions. Following this research, Martin[65] assessed how children of various ages use gender related information to make social judgments. In a study, Martin asked children to predict how much the characters of a story would like a particular toy.

Martin saw that younger children (four years old) relied on sex alone; older children (six years old) took into consideration other variables as well, such as information provided about the characters' interests.

8   CULTURAL RELATIVISM

Different socio-cultural groups have different gender divides.[66] Lorber, for example, noted that American Indians have *men, women, and berdache*; in India there are the *hijra*; [67] in Oman the *xanith*. These are men who behave, dress, and work as women, and are as such treated by society. Other societies that acknowledge a third gender can be found in Alaska (with the *Koniag*), Madagascar (*Tanala*), Nubia (*Mesakin*), and Siberia (*Chukchee*). Lorber also reports the existence of societies within Africa and amongst American Indians which recognise *women with the heart of a man*, who therefore work and live as men.[68] In Albania, there are the *sworn virgins*.[69] In families where a man is lacking, the more robust women take their role, with all that involves.

Feinberg notes: "Writing about his expedition into northeastern Brazil in 1576, Pedro de Magalhaes noted females among the Tupinamba who lived as men and were accepted by other men, and who hunted and went to war. His team of explorers, recalling the Greek Amazons, renamed the river that flowed through that area the *River of Amazons* ".[70] Among the native populations of America, these were considered as 'Two-Spirit people'. According to Feinberg, the French missionary Joseph Francois Lafitau noted in the 1700s that the Two-Spirit people were honoured and regarded as people of a higher order.[71]

Feinberg recounts innumerable instances in which trans people have been present in various societies, and about the way they may have been integrated or ostracised within different social contexts.[72] Feinberg, for example, points out that Joan of Arc was indeed condemned to death not for heresy, but for cross dressing, because she refused, before the Inquisition of the Catholic Church, "to stop dressing in garb traditionally worn by men".[73]

The recognition of different sexes and genders in other societies, and the different reactions, ranging from acceptance to ostracism, has typically been taken as 'proof' that gender is a social convention and not a biological datum. Gross argues that if gender divide was a biological fact one could expect a similar gender divide in all societies.[74] It should be noted that this is not necessarily a valid inference. We have seen that biology allows for a variety of sexes and genders, and yet our society only recognises two. The reverse could be true: that some societies acknowledge more genders for historical and social reasons. What happens in other societies is thus not necessarily an indication that sex and gender are pure social constructs. However, of course, the fact that other societies have recognised or do recognise a more diverse series of sexualities and gender identities should inspire us to reflect upon the conceptual and ethical limits of a rigid dichotomous gender divide.

9   CONCLUSIONS

How gender develops is an issue that many psychologists have investigated. This chapter has shown that the very question is kaleidoscopic: it refers to which biological facts are relevant to formation of gender identity and in what ways; it refers to whether there are social roles that are more or less appropriate to males and females; it refers to the social and cultural variables that shape people's roles within their family/social institutions; it refers to the way children learn, or discover, or create who they are, and so on.

Thus the question as to *what is gender identity* and the question as to *how it is formed (or discovered)* cannot be answered univocally. Like the question *what is gender* cannot be answered univocally because gender is an inherently vague notion, used differently in different research contexts, the question of *what is gender identity* also does not lend itself to an unequivocal answer.

Gender identity is best understood as a fundamental element of a broader notion of who each of us is, as a segment of personal identity. As such, it is unique to each individual, as unique as each of his or her constituent characteristics.

The theoretical and empirical studies reported in this chapter also show that there is not one clear explanation for gender identity, both in 'normal' cases and in 'abnormal' cases. It is conceptually and empirically impossible to answer the question of *how gender develops* and *why some people* have a peaceful gender development and others do not. All processes of gender identification are equally complicated, in the sense that in all cases, even when people do not realise it, gender identity results from an interplay of cultural, familial, biological, and perhaps historical facts that escape lucid analysis and observation. From an epistemological point of view, therefore, there is no reason to distinguish *normal from abnormal* gender identification. All processes are equally complex (or equally simple), equally normal and abnormal, equally ambiguous, equally nonunderstood.

This analysis of empirical studies also shows that absolute deference to one theoretical model can be harmful. No theoretical model has provided a conclusive answer to the questions of what gender identity is and how it develops (and perhaps it could not, as this chapter suggests). Each of these theories probably captures some elements of a complex picture. From a clinical point of view, therefore, caution and scepticism should always be used. In practice this means that whereas, for example, psychoanalysis may help some people, others may be better assisted by medical intervention, others by surgery, and so on.

   A final point: it may be assumed that if a condition is biological in nature, then biological treatment is the choice. If it is psychological or social, then only psychotherapy or social interventions are appropriate. It is therefore tempting to seek the physiological causes of gender dysphoria: a biological explanation may appear to give legitimacy to the condition and to ground a right to access medical treatment otherwise more wholly. This is a *non sequitur*. A condition may have no known somatic cause, but biological treatment may still be clinically and ethically appropriate. I will argue (Chapter 6) that on many occasions it is unethical to withdraw medical treatment from children with gender dysphoria; what is important to stress is that, if this is so, it is *not* necessarily because gender dysphoria has primarily biological causes. The answer to the question of whether transgenders have a right to medical treatment is largely independent of the answer to the question of whether transgenderism is a physiological condition. The conclusions of this chapter, thus, have no bearing upon the normative discourses on entitlement to access medical treatment. We shall return to this point in Chapter 9.

4 What Is 'Gender Identity Disorder'?
Tales of People in Between

1 INTRODUCTION: PINOCCHIO

I will now narrate a revised version of the well known fairy tale *Pinocchio*. Up to a certain point, the quotations are faithful to the original, but soon the story will unfold in a different way.

> *Centuries ago there lived—*
> *"A king!" my little readers will say immediately.*

> *No [. . .] you are mistaken. Once upon a time there was a piece of wood. It was not an expensive piece of wood. Far from it. Just a common block of firewood, one of those thick, solid logs that are put on the fire in winter to make cold rooms cosy and warm. I do not know how this really happened, yet the fact remains that one fine day this piece of wood found itself in the shop of an old carpenter. His real name was Mastro Antonio, but everyone called him Mastro Cherry, for the tip of his nose was so round and red and shiny that it looked like a ripe cherry. As soon as he saw that piece of wood, Mastro Cherry was filled with joy. Rubbing his hands together happily, he mumbled half to himself: "This has come in the nick of time. I shall use it to make the leg of a table." He grasped the hatchet quickly to peel off the bark and shape the wood. But as he was about to give it the first blow, he stood still with arm uplifted, for he had heard a wee, little voice say in a beseeching tone: "Please be careful! Do not hit me so hard!"*
> *What a look of surprise shone on Mastro Cherry's face! His funny face became still funnier. He turned frightened eyes about the room to find out where that wee, little voice had come from and he saw no one! He looked under the bench—no one! He peeped inside the closet—no one! He searched among the shavings—no one! He opened the door to look up and down the street—and still no one! "Oh, I see!" he then said, laughing and scratching his wig. "It can easily be seen that I only thought I heard the tiny voice say the words! Well, well—to work once more."*

He struck a most solemn blow upon the piece of wood. "Oh, oh! You hurt!" cried the same far-away little voice. Mastro Cherry grew dumb, his eyes popped out of his head, his mouth opened wide, and his tongue hung down on his chin.

As soon as he regained the use of his senses, he said, trembling and stuttering from fright: "Where did that voice come from, when there is no one around? Might it be that this piece of wood has learned to weep and cry like a child? I can hardly believe it. Here it is—a piece of common firewood, good only to burn in the stove, the same as any other. Yet—might someone be hidden in it?"

This is how the story of Pinocchio begins. As we all know, Mastro Cherry handed the wood log to Geppetto, who took his tools and began to cut and shape the wood into a Marionette. "What shall I call him?" he said to himself. "I think I'll call him PINOC-CHIO. This name will make his fortune. I knew a whole family of Pinocchi once—Pinocchio the father, Pinocchia the mother, and Pinocchi the children—and they were all lucky. The richest of them begged for his living."

After choosing the name for his Marionette, Geppetto set seriously to work to make the hair, the forehead, the eyes. Fancy his surprise when he noticed that these eyes moved and then stared fixedly at him.

After the eyes, Geppetto made the nose, which began to stretch as soon as it was finished. It stretched and stretched and stretched till it became so long, it seemed endless. Poor Geppetto kept cutting it and cutting it, but the more he cut, the longer grew that impertinent nose.

Next Geppetto made the mouth. He carved a smile on Pinocchio's face, but the more he curved it up, the more the mouth bended down in a line of sorrow. The more Geppetto re-carved, the more the mouth re-bended. Next Geppetto carved the eyes. He made big beautiful eyes, but as he carved their edges pointing up, they turned down, making Pinocchio look more like a Pierrot than a Pinocchio!

As Geppetto eventually got round the idea that his Marionette was somehow alive, he cried: "I am going to make you happy, Son!" Geppetto bought toys for Pinocchio, and fed and dressed him well. Pinocchio's health was good, and yet, as the days and months went by, Pinocchio remained sad. Geppetto did not know what was wrong with his Pinocchio. He bought new toys for him, he took him to the park to play outside with the other children, he even took him to the Marionette's show, to see Arlecchino and Pulcinella and the Fire Eater, just in case he'd enjoy watching other marionettes, and yet. . . Pinocchio's nose continued to grow, and the more Geppetto carved it short, the more it grew; Pinocchio's mouth always bended down, and immense sadness filled in his eyes.

Then, as is well known, Geppetto one day sent Pinocchio to school, so that he could learn and grow up like all other children. He sold his only coat to buy a school book and a copybook for Pinocchio. Pinocchio, who, in our story, was a grateful and obedient child, diligently attended his first day. Geppetto was very excited. He had not had the chance to go to school, and providing education to his son was the best thing he thought he could do for his child.

On that very first day at school, Geppetto couldn't wait till Pinocchio came back to ask how it went. He opened the door wide as he saw Pinocchio strolling back home with his school book under the armpit: "How did it go, Son??"

Seeing his father so excited about the school, Pinocchio did not have the spirit to disappoint him, and thus he said that it all went well. He lied, and his nose grew and grew.

Geppetto took little notice: "You must be tired now," he said. "I will carve your nose small and then you should take a rest". But when, over dinner, Pinocchio looked out the window, in the dark outside he saw his face reflected through the glass, his wooden still face, and his nose grew again, and for the first time he felt a lump in his wooden stomach, a knot in his wooden throat, and it all sat there, because his wooden eyes could not shed a tear of the immense sadness that filled him.

The grief of Pinocchio is that of a child trapped in a wooden body, a body that does not belong to him, that he cannot control, change, and that makes him different to the world he feels he belongs to. His impertinent nose that grows is the insolent nature of a real child, who longs for being who he is, not different, not visible, and not a stranger. Every time he looks at his own face, he sees a monstrosity, a wooden skin that is not human and that is not him. He knows he is a child; his stomach shrinks like all real stomachs must do, his breath and heart pump faster when he is scared or happy, but his eyes cannot even cry, because woods have no tears.

"Something must have gone wrong somewhere"—he thinks—because he knows he is a child, he thinks and feels like a child, and yet he has been given the body of a Marionette. He clasps his hands over his eyes and stands in front of the big mirror: "I am a child, I am a child, I am a child"—he repeats, then counts 1 2 3 in the hope that once he opens up his hands, the spell has gone and he sees flesh reflected back to him. But the wooden log is there to stare at him. "Maybe I don't wish it hard enough". Nobody, not even his father, seems to take notice of the absurdity that wants him trapped into a wooden log.

What's perhaps worse, they all treat him as if nothing ever went wrong; they all treat him as a child. They all accept and praise him and treat him well. There is thus a wrongness of cosmic proportions: an exorcism hems him in a body that does not represent him, and for some occult reason all seem to think that there is nothing strange at having the heart of a boy in the body of a log.

The loneliness of Pinocchio, the forced lie in which Pinocchio has to live, the sense of estrangement and absurdity can perhaps illustrate the solitude experienced by children with gender variance. Pinocchio is not just a rarity, a part of a minority; he is at the edge of humankind.

2   PINOCCHIO . . . TO BE CONTINUED

This revised fairy tale could have continued in many different ways. Pinocchio stopped going to school and followed the Cat and the Fox. They promised to take him to the Fields of Miracles, where there were other marionettes like him, and where marionettes became boys and girls and everything they felt they wanted to be. . . but he had to do things you are not allowed to do at the Field of Miracles, there were no schools or proper jobs there, and one day the police came and took him with them. Or, in another story, Geppetto and the school teacher understand that something is not right in Pinocchio and together decide to knock on the door of the Good Fairy. . . .

There are many endings to the stories of children with atypical gender. Many, unfortunately, do not have a happy finale. Many transgenders are subjected to high degrees of violence and abuse, as the Council of Europe also reminded us in January 2010 and 2011.[1] The United Nations Human Rights Council adopted a resolution on 17 June 2011 expressing concern about violence and discrimination against individuals for reasons of their sexual or gender orientation.[2] Most transgender adolescents and adults have experienced gender dysphoria since early childhood.[3] But many children remain secretive and live in the pain of an unfulfilled existence. Others find acceptance or validation on the street, and here many get entangled in the juvenile justice system. If timely supportive intervention is denied, the outcome for children with gender variance can be grim.

Gender dysphoria is a serious condition which can be associated with a hideous psychological and social sequelae unless proper care is taken on time. In this chapter I will discuss how gender variance manifests itself and use case histories to illustrate the experience of those affected. I will also consider the clinical features of 'Gender Identity Disorder' (GID), as described by the DMS-IV and the ICD-10.

Once the condition is better understood, I will examine the available treatment options (Chapter 5).

3   WHAT IS GENDER DYSPHORIA?

Here are four case histories.

CASE HISTORY 1: JAN MORRIS

I was three or perhaps four years old when I realised that I had been born into the wrong body and should really be a girl. I remember the moment well, and it is the earliest memory of my life.

I was sitting beneath my mother's piano, and her music was falling around me like cataracts, enclosing me as in a cave. The round stumpy legs of the piano were like three black stalactites, and the sound-box was a high dark vault above my head [. . .] On the fact of things it was pure nonsense. I seemed to most people a very straightforward child, enjoying a happy child-hood. I was loved and I was loving, brought up kindly and sensibly, spoiled to a comfortable degree [. . .] by every standard of logic I was patently a boy. I was named James Humphry Morris, male child. I had a boy's body. I wore a boy's clothes.[4]

CASE HISTORY 2: JAMES

James was referred to the Gender Identity Development Service at the age of eight years. At the assessment interviews, he said that since the age of four or five he had very much wished he were a girl. He had been secretly dressing up in his mother's clothes. He liked to play with dolls and cuddly toys and fan-tasised that he was a mother feeding them. He played weddings and liked to be in the role of the bride. At school he wanted to play with girls and avoided rough-and-tumble play or other activities with boys.[5]

CASE HISTORY 3: JERRY

(My mother) went to the trouble of finding two identical dresses—one for me and one for my sister. My sister loved hers. I didn't. Mother put the dress on me, I took it off. My mother put it on me again, and I took it off. She tried again and again, and I took it off again—only this time I cut it up with scissors.[6]

CASE HISTORY 4: ANONYMOUS

Imagine how you would feel if, tomorrow morning, you were to wake up to find yourself in a male body, with a man's voice and a man's face looking back at you from the mirror, with early morning beard and moustache stubble, with no breasts, an Adam's apple, large male feet and hands, a body covered in thick, black hair and a penis and testicles [. . .] Do you think that you'd feel as if you were going crazy? [. . .] This terrible thing has happened to me and it is worse than you could ever imagine (personal communication).

These are four short case histories of children with atypical gender develop-ment. Often gender variance makes its onset at a very young age.[7] In July 2008 the newspaper the *Times* reported the story of Sharon Lane (pseud-onym), a mother who found her twelve-year-old son, Nick, trying to cut off his penis. At the age of five, Nick had declared: "God has made a mistake. I should have been born a girl".[8]

Even those, like Jan Morris, who seek help in adulthood often declare that they had awareness of their condition early on in life. Typically, the accounts provided by sufferers share important similarities. Lewins out-lines these as follows:

a) the long personal history of tension between biological sex and pre-ferred gender or, as many transsexuals put it, having a conviction of being in the wrong body. Katherine Cummings [. . .] eloquently captures this tension: "I can only reiterate the image so often used by transsexuals, that of feeling locked inside a body in which they do not belong, looking through the eyes of that body as they might through the eyeholes of a mask, or from the windows of a cell [. . .]. In the case of a transsexual locked inside a prison of flesh and blood there is a constant ache for emancipation and sense of wonder that no one senses the cries for help from the prisoner within";[9]
b) the awareness and experience of being different as a child, often accompanied by bullying and teasing at school;
c) the psychological struggle to reconcile the conflict between what the mind is demanding and what the body every day seems to be saying;
d) and the negative social responses to a life of overt transsexualism.[10]

Different nomenclature applies to the experience of atypical gender devel-opment. The Diagnostic and Statistical Manual of Mental Disorders (DSM-IV) and the International Classification of Diseases (ICD-10) utilise the term *Gender Identity Disorder*.[11] As I explained previously, I privilege the term *transgenderism*, but I use transsexualism, gender dysphoria, atyp-ical gender identity organisation, and gender variance as interchangeable. Whereas I do not see problems in using all these terms, I have problems with the word 'disorder'. I anticipated in Chapters 2 and 3 that a 'dis-order' presupposes the existence of an 'order', and we have seen that it is not clear what an 'orderly' gender identity development is. In Chapter 8 I will further investigate the epistemological issues relating to the classification of gender dysphoria as pathology. Thus I will use the notion of 'disorder' only in those limited circumstances in which I refer to diagnostic criteria.

GID was first included in the DSM-III in 1980. It is now included in the DSM-IV and in the ICD-10 (F64).[12] There is a category of GID of Child-hood (at F64.2) in the ICD-10 and in the DSM (DSM 302.6). The DSM also includes GID Non Otherwise Specified (NOS).[13] GID will also appear in the DSM-V, due to be published in May 2013, perhaps substituted with the term *gender dysphoria*.[14] Thus, gender dysphoria is formally regarded as a mental illness. I will discuss whether this is epistemologically and ethically appropriate in Chapter 8.

Disorders of gender identification are differentiated from paraphilia of cross dressing or transvestitism (DSM 302.3). In these cases the person is thought to experience sexual arousal and pleasure from wearing clothes of the other sex. Disorders of gender identification are also differentiated from homosexuality, although the trans community sometimes includes gay and lesbian people as well (LGBTs).[15] Homosexuality was included amongst mental illnesses until 1973, when it was replaced by the category of Sexual Orientation Disturbance in the DSM-II and by that of Ego Dystonic Homosexuality in the DSM-III.[16] In 1986 the American Psychiatric Association (APA) decided to remove the category entirely from the DSM.

DSM-IV-TR DIAGNOSTIC CRITERIA FOR GID

A. A strong and persistent cross-gender identification (not merely a desire for any perceived cultural advantages of being the other sex). In children, the disturbance is manifested by four (or more) of the following:

    Repeatedly stated desire to be, or insistence that he or she is, the other sex.

    In boys, preference for cross dressing or simulating female attire; in girls, insistence on wearing only stereotypical masculine clothing.

    Strong and persistent preferences for cross-sex roles in make-believe play or persistent fantasies of being the other sex.

    Intense desire to participate in the stereotypical games and pastimes of the other sex.[17]

    Strong preference for playmates of the other sex.

B. Persistent discomfort with his or her sex or sense of inappropriateness in the gender role of that sex.

C. The disturbance is not concurrent with a physical intersex condition.

D. The disturbance causes clinically significant distress or impairment in social, occupational, or other important areas of functioning.

ICD-10 2007 VERSION OF GID OF CHILDHOOD[18]

A disorder, usually first manifest during early childhood (and always well before puberty), characterised by a persistent and intense distress about assigned sex, together with a desire to be (or insistence that one is) of the other sex. There is a persistent preoccupation with the dress and activities of the opposite sex and repudiation of the individual's own sex. The diagnosis requires a profound disturbance of the normal gender identity; mere tomboyishness in girls or girlish behaviour in boys is not sufficient. GIDs in individuals who have reached or are entering puberty should not be classified here but in F66.

4   CLINICAL DESCRIPTION

GID is described as a "condition in which individuals experience their 'gender identity' as being incongruent with their *phenotype* (the external sexual characteristics of the body)".[19] Broadly speaking, gender dysphoria is defined as "discomfort or distress that is caused by a discrepancy between a person's gender identity and that person's sex assigned at birth (and the associated gender role and/or primary and secondary sex characteristics)".[20] The intensity with which the dysphoria may manifest itself of course varies: some children demonstrate extreme non-conforming behaviours and wishes, and/or severe discomfort with their primary sex characteristics; in others, these features are less marked.

A sufferer narrates: "I found it very difficult to know how to behave as a boy, things that were automatic for other boys, immediate responses that were in keeping with their gender, in-built and natural, weren't like that for me. Even at four I felt outside the equation but I was not sure why".[21] In many, although not in all cases, the discomfort begins early in childhood. In some cases, the child with gender dysphoria—usually manifested in atypical gender role behaviour—will become a homosexual, transvestite, or heterosexual adult. Some sources report that only a small minority of children with atypical gender development will become transsexual (the majority develop homosexual orientation or heterosexual orientation without transvestitism or transsexualism).[22] Others instead contend that the earlier the phenomenon arises, the more rigidly structured it is likely to become during growth.[23] Those experiencing gender variance in adolescence almost invariably go on to experience it in adulthood (see later in this chapter for more detailed information on psychosexual outcome).[24]

Growing in a body that is experienced as inappropriate is for some terrifying and intolerable, and taking whatever step is necessary to express their 'true' identity is for many a life-or-death choice.[25] Typically, children with gender dysphoria experience the first signs of puberty as extremely distressing, "and puberty might have a strong negative effect on their emotional and social functioning, and on their school career".[26]

Many of those born in areas of the world where early treatment and sex change medical interventions are unavailable emigrate clandestinely to countries where they will be able to transition to the other gender; they may become prostitutes in order to pay for reassignment surgery, thus exposing themselves to HIV, STDs, imprisonment, violence, and abuse. Sometimes, in order to survive the cold winter nights on the pavement, they resort to heroin, thus again adopting criminalised behaviours and exposing themselves to life threatening conditions.[27] Even those who do not need to emigrate in order to obtain reassignment treatments (hormonal therapies and surgery) sometimes do not receive timely medical intervention and may get entangled in a dangerous lifestyle while searching for acceptance amongst peers (often in the street) and hormonal treatment from nonmedical sources, such as the illegal market.[28]

That some youths may initiate medical treatment without supervision is a serious concern. Meininger and Remafedi, for example, report that amongst those who decide to take this route, it may be common to share needles with friends. Thirty-one per cent of adult female to male and 80 per cent of adult male to female resort to prostitution as a way of raising money for medical care. There also seems to be evidence that prostitution circles offer to some a validation of their gender identity and a reduction of the stigma and isolation associated with atypical gender identification. One Californian study reports that as many as 63 per cent of the black transgender male to female youths have HIV.[29]

As it will be explained at greater length in the section on the social dimension, transgender people are also particularly at risk of abuse and violence.[30] The long term effects of continued verbal and physical abuse are severe, as we will see shortly.[31] There have been even cases of children killed by their peers because of their atypical gender identity.[32] Transgender adults are also at high risk of violence and murder.[33]

Transgenderism is thus a problem that afflicts not only the individuals concerned and their families; it is an issue of public health as well as a social issue. Gender dysphoria has three dimensions: a psychological, a physical, and a social dimension, which will be explored in the following sections.

5   GENDER DYSPHORIA: A THREE DIMENSIONAL ISSUE

Atypical gender identification has three main and interrelated dimensions: intra-psychic, physical, and social.

5.1   Intra-Psychic Dimension

Gender dysphoria is associated with significant distress. Di Ceglie described the intra-psychic experience of children as follows: "Their interests, their play, their fantasies, their way of moving or talking, their way of relating to friends, or their way of seeing themselves do not fit the body that they have and the way that other people perceive them as a consequence of their bodily appearance. One might say that their psyche lives in a foreign body. [. . .] The child feels driven to live in this confusing and bewildering condition".[34]

In addition, because the child is often aware of not meeting the expectations of others, s/he may experience strong feelings of guilt.[35] For this reason, many remain secretive about their needs and feelings, fearing not only that they will be rejected socially, but also that they will disappoint their significant others.[36] I will return to this later in this chapter.

During adolescence, the unease becomes more distressing. As puberty progresses, transgender boys will develop breasts, may start to menstruate, and sometimes become frustrated by their small stature. Transgender girls' voices may deepen, they may grow beards and prominent Adam's apples, experience erections, and became taller than most other women. These experiences are profoundly humiliating for transgender youths. The uncertainty over the sense of self, and the secrecy and isolation that often accompany young people through their atypical gender development, may lead to psychological disintegration. Children and adolescents with atypical gender development appear to be at high risk of suicide.[37]

Not only denigration, but also open violence is sometimes used against people, including children and adolescents, with unusual gender expressions (see Section 5.3). Clearly, violence is the extreme manifestation of psychological and social rejection of the phenomenon.[38] In this context, isolation and secrecy appear appropriate forms of self-defence.

5.2 Physical Dimension

Gender dysphoria does not generally cause physical alterations, and it is not caused by a known alteration in physical functioning. Children with gender dysphoria generally develop 'normally', in accordance with what is considered to be their biological sex. However, gender identity is not congruent, or fully congruent, with the body and with the social roles that are attached to the sex of assignment.

In some cases, gender dysphoria appears in concomitance with other conditions, which might alter sex development (DSDs—see Chapter 2). In these cases, as we have seen before, the sexual development of the individual might be ambiguous, for example, if the genitalia are ambiguous or if enzymes prevent complete virilisation in biological males or if chromosomal anomalies are present. Ghosh and Walker have provided a clear account of DSDs and of their relationship with gender dysphoria.[39] As they explain, gender dysphoria should not be confused with these other conditions. Although sometimes they appear together, typically gender dysphoria sufferers have a clear phenotypical appearance congruent with the sex assigned at birth, but incongruent gender identity. De Vries et al. also studied the relationship between intersex conditions and gender dysphoria, and warned clinicians not to attach too much value to neurophysiological factors when approaching gender variance.[40]

The physical dimension of gender dysphoria encompasses instead a series of important physical changes for those who decide to transition, partly or completely, to the other gender. I will discuss the physical sequelae associated with gender treatment in Chapter 5. It is important to anticipate here that when the problem is identified early and treatment begins early, severe mutilating surgery can be avoided and much better physical outcomes can obviously be achieved. Those who transition later in life are less likely to obtain a fully satisfactory appearance, as when changes have taken place due to 'natural' growth, some of them are irreversible or only partly reversible via hormonal and surgical treatment.

5.3   Social Dimension

Gender dysphoria is also, in a profound way, a social issue, at least in two ways. First, gender dysphoria is, to an important extent, shaped by social categories and stereotypes about gender. As we have seen in Chapters 2 and 3, gender studies have argued that 'women' and 'men' are to an important degree socially constructed notions and entities. To the extent that they are right, the same must apply to the transgenders.

Not surprisingly, gender dysphoria is particularly stressful within certain socio-cultural contexts. Western societies have struggled to contemplate gender ambiguity or differences as one of the many, normal paths open to individuals, and the psychological distress experienced by the sufferer and the family is partly due to the social difficulty of accepting the reality of 'alternative ways' of being. In societies where the gender divide is not as rigid, people in fact appear to suffer less, and some forms of transgenderism can even be encouraged or praised socially in some societies (see also Chapter 3, Section 9).[41]

Notably, even within Western societies, the referral rates for GID appear less where there is greater tolerance of cross-gender behaviours. For example, in the Netherlands, where social tolerance is higher, the percentage of referrals between ages three and six years is 13 per cent, compared to Toronto, which has a percentage rate of 40.5 per cent. The difference becomes more pronounced for ages three to five years—2.3 per cent in Utrecht compared to 22.6 per cent in Toronto.[42]

Second, people with gender dysphoria, including children and adolescents, are exposed to bullying, abuse, and denigration, as well as to open physical violence or even murder.[43] The child, it is reported, "will confront varying degrees of curiosity or teasing from peers and adults".[44] S/he is at risk for social isolation and ostracism, violence, and recurrent threats to self-esteem. The child's parents may also face stigmatisation and may themselves feel insecure, embarrassed, and conflicted, leading to punitive and critical responses to their child".[45] According to one study, children and adolescents with gender dysphoria are regularly subject to rejection, discrimination, and abuse.[46] Homophobic bullying in schools is common in the UK.[47] Of the lesbian/gay/bisexual/transgender (LGBT) youths, 89.2 per cent experience verbal bullying; 17.6 per cent are physically assaulted for reasons related to their gender/sexual orientation.[48] One study conducted in Philadelphia also reports that 96 per cent of transgender youths reported being verbally harassed, 83 per cent being physically harassed, and that 75 per cent dropped out of school.[49] Another study conducted in the UK suggests that about 40 per cent of transgender people experienced verbal abuse at school, 30 per cent threatening behaviour, 25 per cent physical abuse, and 4 per cent sexual abuse, and that 25 per cent had been bullied by their teachers. The study reports greater verbal abuse for gay schoolchildren. In public space, 19 per cent had experienced verbal abuse, 10 per cent threatening behaviour, 5 per cent physical abuse, and 2 per cent sexual abuse.[50] Other studies show increased likelihood of homelessness in LGBT youths, high rates of verbal and physical abuse in school, increased likelihood of substance abuse and hepatitis B and C, as well as depression and other mental health concerns.[51]

H., a transgender girl (female to male) aged sixteen at the time she gave this statement, illustrates the sort of abuse that a young transgender may need to endure for reasons relating to his or her diversity: "Many," she wrote, "are ignorant and cruel and they shout out things like, 'Girl with a cock', 'There's the he/she/it', 'Tranny boy', and other names. On my way to school, people shout similar comments from their cars, because of the way I look. I want this school to be the last place that this happens to me. When I leave school, to go to University, or to get a job, I want to be able to keep my private life private; this is nobody else's business".[52]

This type of response to atypical gender has severe long term effects on the child's welfare.[53] Children who are victims of homophobic bullying are five times more likely than other students to fail to attend schools and twice as likely not to pursue further education.[54] Substance abuse, homelessness, prostitution, HIV infection, self-harm, depression, anxiety,[55] and suicide[56] are also included among the results of homophobic bullying.[57]

The threefold distress to which children and adolescents with gender issues are exposed (intra-psychic, physical, and social) makes life unbearable to many of them.[58] A study by Clements-Nolle et al. found that as many as 32 per cent of trans youths attempted suicide.[59]

6 EPIDEMIOLOGY AND PSYCHOSEXUAL OUTCOME

According to one study, in the Netherlands 1 in 11.900 males and 1 in 30.400 females meet the criteria for GID.[60] According to another study, the number of transsexuals in the UK may range between one in one hundred people and one in twenty.[61] A 2009 study reports that prevalence at the time in the UK was twenty per one hundred thousand,[62] of whom 80 per cent assigned as boys at birth (male to female trans) and 20 per cent as girls (female to male trans).

The incidence and prevalence of gender dysphoria in children and adolescents have not been established with certainty.[63] The prevalence *of cross-gender behaviour*, according to a study, is considerable and significantly higher in girls than in boys: 2.6 to 6 per cent for young boys and 5 to 12 per cent for young girls (this difference in sex ratio decreases as children enter adolescence). Interestingly, however, it appears that more boys are referred to clinics (overall ratio between 3.8:1 and 4.7:1 depending on the clinic). The difference in referral rates may be a function of some unknown biological predisposition to gender variance in boys than in girls.[64] However, the higher prevalence of cross-gender behaviour in girls, reported earlier, induces one to think that the difference in sex ratio may relate to greater social tolerance of cross-gender behaviour in girls than in boys.[65] In other words, 'tomboyiness' is more acceptable than 'sissiness'.[66]

A steady increase in referral rates has also been observed.[67] Over the last ten years, the UK Tavistock and Portman Clinic, the only children service in the UK, has seen the number of referrals rise from fifteen to between fifty and sixty per annum.[68] A 2009 report suggests that there are around eighty-four children referred to gender identity services in the UK every year, compared to fifteen hundred referred to adult clinics.[69] These numbers seem consistent across the countries.[70] This means that, on average, each clinic will see at least about one or two new children a week.

The age of onset of gender dysphoria may vary. As we have seen at the beginning of this chapter, young children may begin to express their gender in an atypical manner. Yet how many of these children will become transsexual adults is debated. A study conducted by the Gender Identity Research and Education Society (GIRES) in the UK suggests that it is unknown in how many prepubertal children with gender dysphoria the condition eventually remits. However, if the condition persists after the onset of puberty, it is most likely to continue in adulthood.[71]

Wallien and Cohen-Kettenis reported, in 2008, that 27 per cent of their total group of gender dysphoric prepubertal children they saw were 'persisters': they were persistently dysphoric at the time of follow up, in adolescence.[72] They also found a higher rate of persistence in girls than in boys: 50 per cent of the gender dysphoric girls were persisters. These data are consistent with those provided by Zucker and Bradley,[73] but higher than those illustrated in other studies.[74] Zucker makes a cautious conclusion from these studies: only a minority of children with gender dysphoria are persisters. The majority of boys will become homosexual, and the majority of girls are equally likely to develop homosexual or heterosexual orientation. "From these data", Zucker continues, "then, it is apparent that there is not one 'natural history' for GID in children: some children show a persistence in their gender dysphoria, whereas a large number show a clear desistance".[75] Importantly, Wallien and Cohen-Kettenis warn that "the psychosexual differentiation of children with GID is more variable than what the early studies suggested".[76]

Of course, this raises the question of how clinicians may predict whether a child is a persister or a desister. Wallien and Cohen-Kettenis argue that it is likely that "only children with extreme gender dysphoria are future sex reassignment applicants, whereas the children with less persistent and intense gender dysphoria are future homosexuals or heterosexuals without GID. However, none of the follow up studies have as yet provided evidence for this supposition".[77] In particular, persisters in their study were more likely to meet all the DSM-IV criteria for GID, and they presented more severe cross-gender behaviour and gender dysphoria.[78]

This also raises an issue of how children should be treated medically. Wallien and Cohen-Kettenis write: "If one was certain that a child belongs to the persisting group, interventions with gonadotropin-releasing hormone (GnRH) analogues to delay puberty could even start before puberty rather than after the first pubertal stages, as now often happens. The possibility of identifying the persisters in childhood would also be helpful, if treatments would be available to prevent the intensive and drastic hormonal and surgical treatments these children face in adolescence and adulthood".[79]

At the moment the way the child reacts to the first pubertal changes is still used as a part of diagnosis.[80] Zucker notes that there are three general approaches to gender dysphoria in children: according to one, transgenderism and transsexualism are 'bad outcomes', and therefore therapy aims at lessening the degree of cross-gender behaviour; a second approach makes no attempt to 'correct' cross-gender behaviour, but is also wary of not encouraging it. A third approach is more interventionist, and encourages Real Life Experience or even puberty suppressant medication when there is evidence of strong and persistent dysphoria.

I will discuss the clinical approaches to gender variance in children in Chapter 5. It is important here to begin to mention different approaches as they may affect the rates of persistence and desistance. For example, it can be asked whether "the rate of persistence be higher among those parents and therapists who facilitate an early gender role and gender transition than among those parents and therapists who attempt to lessen the childhood expression of gender dysphoria [. . .]. A second important question is whether these different therapeutic approaches will result in different or distinct long term outcomes with regard to the child's more general psychosocial and psychiatric adjustment".[81]

These questions have not yet been answered. What seems to emerge is that children, from a very young age, express their gender uniquely. Many will adopt, at some point during their development, what may appear to be 'cross-gender' behaviours, but then move on to broadly identify themselves with the assigned gender. If the situation persists at a pubertal stage, there is a greater likelihood that medical and psychological care may be needed.

7   AETIOLOGY

With regard to the aetiology of atypical gender development, (perhaps not surprisingly) no cause has been found. There is instead a variety of theories about gender dysphoria. I offer here only a brief account of these and will make some comments later.

First, we should mention *psychological theories*. The assumption, within this paradigm, is that gender dysphoria is caused by a psychopathology or a pathology in the family.[82] Transsexualism has thus been described in terms of narcissistic disorder, a perversion, or a defence against separation anxiety.[83] Often, based on the assumption that the family plays a fundamental role in the formation of gender identity in the child, the family is held responsible (or even blamed) for the child's condition. These assumptions are obviously speculative and sometimes even conceptually flawed. Regarding psychopathology as the cause of gender dysphoria is circular, and regarding family influences as responsible for the phenomenon is somewhat redundant: clearly the significant others, as we have seen in previous chapters, contribute to the formation of gender identity; however, it is unclear which influences produce what and why some children respond to those in one way whereas others do not. Thus, the family hypothesis remains unsubstantiated and, to an important extent, question begging.

Observations of children treated for those intersex conditions that involve ambiguous genitalia show that gender identity is not always coherent with genital appearance.[84] In these cases, it has been common practice to reduce the genitalia, surgically, to an unambiguous female appearance and to raise the children as girls, and, in addition, to give hormonal support consistent with this reassignment at a later stage. As we have seen in Chapter 3, this is not always successful, and cases where the individual reverts to an apparently innate, indelible gender identity demonstrate that gender cannot always be moulded by upbringing and even by surgery. This seems to imply that, similarly, atypical gender identification may be independent of upbringing and may be well beyond the parents' power.

Second, there are the *biological theories*,[85] searching for the causes of gender dysphoria and cross-gender behaviour in the brain structures,[86] prenatal hormones, or genetics.[87] Genetic studies have shown higher concordance rates of gender variance in twins. However, it is not clear whether these studies involve monozygotic twins or dizygotic twins. Moreover, in order to offer more conclusive evidence, genetic studies should be conducted on monozygotic twins raised separately. These studies have not been performed yet. Thus there seems to be no conclusive evidence of genetic or endocrinological[88] causes of gender dysphoria and cross-gender behaviour.[89] However, there seems to be evidence that some biological factors may be involved in transgenderism. Kreukels and Cohen-Kettenis write:

> In the central portion of the bed nucleus of the stria terminalis and the interstitial nuclei 3 and 4 of the anterior hypothalamus, a sex reversal has been found in the volume and number of neurons in male to female transsexuals and a female to male transsexual.[90] Neuroimagining studies indicate that the microstructure pattern of white matter in untreated female to male transsexuals was more similar to the usual pattern in men, and that the gray matter volume of the putamen in untreated

male to female transsexuals had more resemblance to the volume usually seen in women.[91] In addition, cerebral activation patterns in transsexuals before treatment seem to share more features with those of the experienced gender than those of their biological sex. These patterns were observed during the processing of pheromones, and while participants viewed erotic film excerpts. Finally, differences have been found within the cortical network between male to female transsexuals (both before and during hormonal treatment) and control males while the participants are engaged in mental rotation tasks. In addition to the brain studies, findings from behavioural and genetic studies indicate that a genetic component in gender development can not be ruled out, and polymorphism in genes related to sex steroids have been found to differ between transsexual and nontranssexual groups; however, some additional studies have not found support for such polymorphism. Overall, these observations are in line with our clinical experience that GID in adolescents and adults is extremely resistant to change.[92]

7.1 Some Reflections

The search for the causes of a phenomenon, in this case, of gender variance, is a laudable effort. The attempt to understand a condition is linked to the attempt to understand why that condition occurs and how it could be best dealt with.

However, the very questions as to *what causes gender variance* or *why some children develop equivocal gender* need to be understood. It is in particular necessary to clarify what type of answer one wants, and what one is looking for, in posing that question.

When one asks *why this is happening, what caused this*, one probably wants to find a solution to the problem. The interest, therefore, is not merely speculative. The question of aetiology is important mainly for its normative and clinical implications. In other words, understanding the causes of a condition could improve the treatment options or even legitimise them (at least apparently). It may seem that if, for example, it turns out that gender dysphoria is caused by, say, prenatal hormonal exposure, this legitimises the classification of gender dysphoria as an endocrinological disorder, rather than a psychiatric disorder, and may validate the use of hormonal treatment to help the sufferers. If the causes of gender variance are psychological, then perhaps treatment should be based on psychotherapy/group therapy/family therapy, or psychiatric treatment. The question about the causes is in an important way a question about the appropriate modalities of intervention.

But this is a much more vacillating perspective than it looks. If, say, GID is a purely psychological condition, then one may argue, mere psychological treatment is clinically and ethically appropriate, all medical treatment should be avoided. Similarly, if, say, GID appeared to depend on dysfunctional prenatal hormonal exposure, one may argue that GID is then a primarily endocrinological disorder, and this may legitimise the use of endocrinological treatment: *but to what purpose?* The question remains open as to what is a good outcome, and the search for causes seems to hide, sometimes, the implicit goals that one thinks are appropriate in these cases. Stressing how GID is a psychological condition seems to hide an understated assumption that transsexualism is a bad outcome, and that psychological interventions can revert the psychological disorder, causing the person to identify with the wrong gender (we have seen an example of this in the discussion of Freud's approach in Chapter 3).

But also, say that GID appeared to be an endocrinological disorder, one may argue that *therefore* endocrinological treatment is clinically and ethically appropriate: but should this treatment be given *to allow the person to change gender*? This would be rather peculiar, because generally the disorder is treated with the aim of moderating its effects, and not with the aim of amplifying them: if transsexualism is the result of a disorder, then the aim should be to cure the disorder and revert transsexualism. For example, when hormonal treatment for retarded growth is provided, this is given in order to revert the course of the disorder, not to propel it. In the case of transgenderism, hormonal treatment that allows the person to cross gender would be given in stark contradiction with the usual goals of medicine. There is thus the impression that the search for the causes of a condition wants to legitimise the goals that one already has in mind, but one has to be careful not to incur contradictions that could, in effect, bring about results opposite to those one wants to achieve.

As I will argue further in Chapter 9, instead, the aetiology itself says little about how people should be treated and why. In other words, the aetiology *per se* has scarce normative or clinical value, contrary to what one may think. There may be conditions whose causes are unknown, but it is known that a certain medical treatment is helpful. For example, the causes of bipolar disorder are unknown, but it is known that lithium carbonate may be helpful. The causes of myalgic fibrosis are unknown, but it is known that dopamine reuptakers may ease the discomfort. In fact, sometimes the causes become clearer given that a treatment helps. The case of Parkinson's disease is an illustration of this. It was noted that dopamine inhibitors reduced psychotic symptoms in patients with paranoid schizophrenia. However, it was also noted that when dopamine levels dropped under a certain threshold due to excessive doses of medication, patients with schizophrenia developed tremors and other symptoms of Parkinson's disease. It was thus speculated that dopamine reuptakers could ease the symptoms of Parkinson's disease. Dopamine is now used as a standard treatment for Parkinson's disease, and Parkinson's disease is now explained in terms of decreased levels of dopamine. This illustrates how sometimes it is the efficacy of a therapy that may reveal something about the causes of a condition.

In many cases, the moral justification for treatment lies in the fact that treatment is likely to alleviate suffering. The fact that the causes of the disease are unknown is secondary or morally and clinically irrelevant. There are even cases in which medical treatment is administered in absence of pathology: pain relief in labour, contraception, and other infertility treatments are provided sometimes even if the condition is not pathological. I will discuss these issues at greater length in Chapters 8 and 9. Whereas the aetiology of gender development is unknown, this is no reason to worry about the clinical and ethical legitimacy of healthcare.

Moreover, as suggested in Chapters 2 and 3, the question as to the causes of gender variance may be somehow misguiding. Of course, this is not to undermine the value of scientific knowledge about human development. Yet, it should be recognised that all forms of gender development are the result of a combination of factors, including biological, social, and cognitive factors. To ask 'what has gone wrong' with gender dysphoric people is to assume that something has actually gone right in other cases, and this is not necessarily a sound assumption. A 'dis-order', as said before, presupposes the existence of an 'order', but what this 'order' is and of what it consists is not clear (nor it can be, on reflection).

KEY POINTS

- Gender variance is characterised by a profound sense of mismatch between one's biological body and one's sense of gender identity.
- In children, is manifested with a repeatedly stated desire to be, or insistence that s/he is, of the other sex (see DSM and ICD for more).
- It is thought that adolescents experiencing gender dysphoria typically will experience it in adulthood.
- Gender variance is typically accompanied by distress in social functioning.
- 89.2 per cent of LGBT youths in the UK experience verbal bullying.
- 17.6 per cent are physically assaulted for reasons related to their gender/sexual orientation.
- Lack of education, substance abuse, homelessness, prostitution, HIV infection, self-harm, depression, anxiety, and suicide are also included among the results of homophobic bullying.
- In societies where the gender divide is not as rigid, people appear to suffer less.

KEY POINTS: EPIDEMIOLOGY AND AETIOLOGY

- There are no clear epidemiological data.
- Specialist clinics see on average one/two new children per week.
- The number of transsexuals (including adults and children) in the UK may range between one in one hundred people and one in twenty.[93]
- The age of onset of gender dysphoria may vary.
- No single cause/set of causes has been found.

8   PINOCCHIO AND THE UGLY DUCKLING

Near Pinocchio and Geppetto's modest house, there was a park with a lake and trees and flowers and birds and geese and ducks. "Before I do my homework, I will stroll around the lake on my own for a while", thought Pinocchio. "Dad", he cried. "I will be back for my homework and dinner". "All right, Son, look after yourself". Pinocchio headed off. He sat on the bench by the lake. There he saw a family of ducks. He jumped off the bench, when he noticed a black duckling! *"I have never seen a black duckling before!!!" he thought. Bewildered, Pinocchio followed the ducks around the lake, observing them. Mother duck was ahead of a group of seven ducklings. All of them were fluffy and yellow and grouped together whistling about happily. And a little farther away, left behind, a little greyish duckling tried to keep up the pace, making clumsy hops and funny whistles. As they swam about in the lake, Pinocchio was hearing the other birds and animals around the lake staring or even laughing about this ugly, clumsy duckling: "Another joke of nature", Pinocchio mumbled, "exactly like me. . . ."*

Every day, Pinocchio went to the lake, to look for the black duckling. The black duckling was sad and stubborn. Everybody made fun of him, of his clumsy attempts at doing what his brothers and sisters were doing, flying, swimming, hunting.. . . He looked at his wings with a puzzled gaze in his eyes, as if wondering why his wings had the colour of the bottom of the lake!

"Hey Duckling!" finally Pinocchio got the courage to call. The little black duckling looked around. "Hey Duckling, it's me, Pinocchio.. . ." "You talking to me?" "Yes, you. Come to the side, I want to talk to you but I can't swim.. . ." The little duckling made himself closer to Pinocchio, slightly worried. Nobody ever talked to him from outside the lake. "What's your name?", asked Pinocchio. "Not sure, they call me the black duckling". "Ah. . . are they your brothers and sisters?" "Yes, they can do lots of stuff, like they can swim and they are learning to fly and they can hunt.. . ."

From then onwards, every day Pinocchio went to the lake, and he and the black duckling became best friends.

One day, however, Pinocchio could no longer see the black duckling in the lake. He ran all around the lake, but there was no sign of his friend. Then he started calling his name loudly. A young swan came close to him then: "Hey Pinocchio, why are you crying so loud?" "I have lost my best friend, have you seen the black duckling? He is my best and only friend". "Pinocchio!" The swan laughed. Pinocchio stared at him, bewildered and suspicious. "Yes Pinocchio, it is true. One day everyone grew white and, like mom, like a real duck. . . but that day they were all bemused when they looked at me. I didn't understand what was happening, so I walked up to the shore and looked at myself on the lake. I nearly lost my bearings when I saw a swan! My surprise was such that I jumped back and fell on my bum! And since then I live on the other side of the lake, where my true relatives are.. . .." He looked at the big swans, and one of them waved with a smile at Pinocchio. Pinocchio made a small bow, with a mixture of worry and consternation.

And here we realise something that, paradoxically, was quite tragic for Pinocchio. Unlike the black duckling. . . beg your pardon, the swan, Pinocchio had not been ridiculed by anyone; he had not been rejected or neglected or made fun of. He had all the love and support that any child could desire. . . or that any puppet could desire. Ironically, this made things even harder for him. Geppetto had no idea of what was going on inside him, and, if he had told Geppetto about how he felt, he'd be shocked, sad, he'd feel betrayed, he'd feel as if it was his fault to have made him this way.. . . Pinocchio could not do this to his dad, who loved him so dearly. The ducks had ignored, neglected, and even ridiculed the black duckling. He could then turn away from them with little regret. But Pinocchio could not turn away from his father: he could not even suggest to his father how wrong and sad he was, how desperate he was. . . .

In this revised fairy tale, two stories of diversity meet. The black duckling and Pinocchio become best friends by virtue of their diversity. However, the duckling was the victim of an error: it was a case of egg swapping. Once the mistake was amended, the duckling could find his 'real' place and be accepted by his peers. The mistake that condemns Pinocchio to his diversity, instead, is not circumstantial; it is mysterious, it is inherent to his own nature, and it cannot be amended. He will never be able to find his own place or his own peers because his peers do not exist. He will be able to have peace only once his body transitions (should this be possible) *beyond his birth*. Until then, Pinocchio is at the borders of humankind.

This is the feeling that many transgenders may have. Lack of identification with a group of belonging may render the condition extremely difficult to conceptualise and communicate. The revised tale also wants to bring attention to the drama experienced by those children who are actually well cared for by their families. Children with gender dysphoria often have supportive families. There is in fact no evidence, as we have seen, that gender variance is caused by dysfunctions in the family. This can paradoxically make the predicaments of gender variance more complex, as the child may wish to protect his/her family from the distress s/he is experiencing, and may not wish to give to the family what s/he may fear is a disappointment. This of course does not mean that a supportive environment promotes secrecy and isolation in the child, but brings attention to the fact that many of these children may find it difficult to express their dis-ease in awareness of the vast implications that this may have not only within their own lives, but in the lives of those close to them.

The following testimonial further illustrates this. This is offered by a transgender who decided to never seek medical treatment. He married, had children, and decided to stick to his male role and responsibilities for the sake of his family.

> [The problem with gender is] not just about you, it is about those you love and the social environment you have to live in. It takes tremendous courage to wear your soul on your shoulders and go and show the 'real' you to the world. Even more so to your parents, who have dreams and aspirations that are in line with physical gender [. . .] The fear of rejection, bullying, hatred are very real even with family for most of these children. The fear of total dismissal of how you feel can be even worse [. . .] In the end you make a choice, you live a life where you face untold difficulty to be who you are and perhaps have to give everyone and everything up to achieve that. Or you live in the shadows never achieving peace and living a life that can never truly be fulfilled.[94]

9   CONCLUSIONS

This chapter has explored what gender dysphoria is thought to be and how it manifests itself, with a particular attention paid to children and adolescents. Incidence, prevalence, and aetiology have been discussed.

This chapter also explored the psychological, physical, and social sequelae associated with atypical gender development and the difficulties that those with atypical gender development may experience, especially in Western societies.

I have wanted to express this condition, which often affects children, in a way that even children could understand, thus by referring to well known children stories which may capture some of the aspects of atypical gender identification and can help to make sense of it.

In the next chapter I will discuss what can be done for children and adolescents suffering from atypical gender development.

5 Available Treatments for Transgender Children and Adolescents

And for everybody, the others' pain is a pain in half.

(F. De André and I. Fossati, 'Disamistade', 1996)[1]

1 INTRODUCTION

In this chapter I discuss the treatments that can be offered to children and adolescents with gender dysphoria.[2] I will firstly offer a brief overview of the treatment approaches available, explaining the underlying theoretical assumptions and treatment goals. Later in this chapter I will focus mainly on the so called 'combined approach', which involves the use of medication. As I will show, this is the most promising option for children and adolescents, and also somehow the most controversial. I will examine the ethical and legal issues that these treatments raise in Chapters 6 and 7. I will argue throughout the book that intervening with medication with young transgenders may be the best option; medical treatment can be a valuable help to gender minorities, and it may be unethical to deny it. Transgendersim is not necessarily a bad outcome, not necessarily a tendency to be counteracted by the healthcare profession. I have so far stressed that transgenderism is not necessarily to be considered as a pathological ill adjustment to the 'natural' (and hence healthy) body; gender development encompasses a variety of forces that shape one's identity in a unique manner. There is not one healthy and one pathological way in which gender develops, and between the two 'standard' (and fictional) notions of *male and female* there posits a wide range of legitimate states in between. In some cases, individuals need medical assistance in order to express more fully who they are. Before moving to the conceptual, ethical, and legal issues surrounding provision of gender treatment to minors, it is important to clarify what these treatments may consist of.

It should be noted that literature on treatment for GID mostly consists of case reports and treatment protocols.[3] No randomised research studies have been conducted, and this makes it difficult to draw conclusions relating to the most successful therapy. The earliest interventions have been oriented at modifying the child's behaviour.[4] It is to this that I now turn.

2 BEHAVIOURAL THERAPY

One of the first approaches used with children with atypical gender identification has been behavioural therapy.[5] The aim of behavioural therapies was to reduce cross-gender behaviours and strengthen same sex behaviour. The assumption here was that the child acquires the 'problematic' behaviour within the (probably dysfunctional) environment in which s/he is raised. The child learns inappropriate responses, and the main goal of therapy is to allow the child to reduce cross-gender behaviour. As in all behavioural therapies, the methods used consisted mainly in providing positive reinforcements for same sex behaviours and negative reinforcements for cross-gender behaviours. Parents were taught how to use these tokens to assist the child at home.

One of the major objections that this approach soon received, beyond the usual criticisms towards behavioural therapies, which stress how these therapies focus on the behaviour somewhat disregarding the reasons for that behaviour, was that it is unethical to prevent the development of one person's gender and sexuality. Behavioural therapy implies, in other words, that cross-gender behaviour and homosexuality are types of deviance, and that it is good to try and amend or prevent them. A similar criticism, as we are now going to see, has been moved against the psychoanalytic approaches.

3 PSYCHOLOGICAL THERAPIES[6]

It is widely recognised that, even when medical treatment is deemed appropriate, this should ideally be accompanied by psychotherapy and family involvement (see for example the guidelines by the Endocrine Society reported in Box 5.3).[7] However, psychotherapy alone does not seem to offer sufficient help to transgender children and adolescents.[8] Whereas there is high emotional distress in these youths, and higher levels of anxiety are noted than in control groups,[9] it seems that emotional distress is a consequence of their gender identity rather than its cause.[10]

There are many different types of psychotherapy: among these are the psychodynamic therapies (based on the psychoanalytic tradition), the cognitive therapy, the Gestalt therapy, the family therapy, the systemic therapy, the cognitive-behavioural therapy, and the transactional therapy, just to mention a few. These approaches differ significantly both in treatment goals, modalities of interaction, and length. The use of psychotherapy is generally recommended to transgenders, but it raises important ethical issues. For example, implicit in the psychoanalytic approach is the assumption that either the individual psychodynamics or the dysfunctions in the family are responsible for cross-gender feelings and behaviours, and that the therapeutic goal is to *resolve* the unconscious conflicts that led up to those feelings and behaviours. There has been a proliferation of cases analysed and 'cured' with psychoanalytic and psychodynamic therapies.[11] As we saw in Chapter 3, Freud's original idea on gender development was that lack of 'proper' sex orientation and gender identification depends on an unresolved Oedipal conflict. Although psychoanalytic and psychodynamic studies provide important information on the relationship between child and family, thus helping to interpret those family dynamics that may be significant in these cases or to help the family to cope with gender variance, the main problem, both conceptual and ethical, of this approach is that gender variance is considered as a dysfunction or the result of a dysfunction, and that a good outcome is one in which cross-gender behaviour is reduced or eliminated.[12]

My arguments so far gesture towards the conclusion that any such assumption is misplaced: a good outcome is one in which the person can flourish and experience their gender with ease, whatever that may be. Whether this is achieved by acquiring congruence with the external phenotypical appearance, by changing that appearance, or by living in gender nomadism or in *in between* states is morally irrelevant and should be clinically irrelevant as well. Whatever can assist the child in achieving a prosperous and happy life is, at least in principle, ethically good, whether this is psychotherapy or medical therapy.

Psychotherapy can certainly assist the child and the family of the transgender child, but it may be opportune that the assumptions and goals be made explicit, in order for the patients to be able to make an informed choice as to whether or not they can share them, or, eventually, negotiate assumptions and goals that are agreeable to them.

Some individuals may integrate their atypical gender feelings into the gender role they were assigned at birth: they may therefore not need to alter their body with medication. Other people may find a way of expressing their perceived gender without medical treatment, and that will be sufficient for them to be comfortable. In other cases, medical intervention or even surgery may be necessary. What is clear is that treatment for gender dysphoria needs to be individualised, and it should be recognised that transgender children and adolescents usually will need a broad range of interventions in order to express more fully who they are. Psychotherapy should thus be used to help individuals to explore their gender concerns, with the overarching goal of achieving long term comfort with their gender identity. It should not be considered as a way of altering a person's perceived gender.[13]

4   TREATMENT FOR PARENTS AND GROUP THERAPIES

Treatment for parents involves working with the parents, understanding their gender ideology, and helping them to develop a positive relationship with their child. According to this approach, working with the parents is essential to resolution of the gender identity issues. The aim of this therapy, first designed by Meyer-Bahlburg,[14] is to reduce cross-gender behaviour.[15]

Group therapy, instead, has historically been offered to children and adolescents with various therapeutic goals.[16] In some approaches, the main goal is to reduce cross-gender behaviour, whereas in others it is to accept the child and attempt to minimise the social effects associated with cross-gender behaviour. There are no long term follow up studies for parents' therapies and group therapies. However, clinical experience shows that there is no evidence that attempts to modify cross-gender behaviours and gender dysphoria are successful.[17]

5   ETHERAPY AND DISTANCE COUNSELLING

The World Professional Association for Transgender Health (WPATH) includes online therapy (etherapy) and distance counselling among the range of interventions that may be made available to transgenders. This type of therapy may be particularly useful to those who have difficulties in accessing competent psychotherapeutic treatment. Etherapy or distance counselling may counteract the isolation and marginalisation that some transgenders may experience, especially in areas in which specialised healthcare provision is lacking. However, there is insufficient evidence based data to establish the advantages and disadvantages of this approach for this category of patients, and therefore caution is urged. Some of the possible advantages and risks are discussed by Fraser and by WPATH.[18]

6   COMBINED APPROACHES

A combined approach includes administration of psychotherapy, social intervention, family work, and medical treatment. In the early 1990s Domenico Di Ceglie and colleagues were among the first in the UK to propose such an approach at the Tavistock and Portman Clinic in London.[19] In the combined approach, the child is first assessed by a multidisciplinary team. Where the extent of gender dysphoria is significant, Di Ceglie suggested that temporary administration of puberty suppressant medications, later cross sex hormones, and, eventually, surgery in adulthood may be appropriate. This approach will be analysed in further detail later in this chapter.[20]

Another important combined treatment protocol is the one offered at the University Medical Center in Amsterdam.[21] This is similar to the one proposed in the UK by Di Ceglie. First the child is assessed by a multidisciplinary team of specialists, including endocrinologists, psychologists, and psychiatrists. Both the child and family are evaluated. The main aim of this approach is to release distress and improve the child's quality of life. The aim, thus, is not to reduce cross-gender behaviour, but to understand it and help the child to overcome his/her vulnerabilities.

Importantly, this approach does not rule out, and indeed contemplates, the administration of medications, such as puberty suppressant medications. As purely psychotherapeutic interventions do not prove to be highly successful in general (although of course they may be successful in individual cases), and as combined approaches appear much more promising, as we shall shortly see, in the rest of this chapter I will concentrate on these. I will provide an account of combined treatments available and of their known risks and benefits. In the next chapter, I will discuss some of the most important ethical concerns raised by these treatments.

7   THREE STAGED INTERVENTIONS

Combined therapy for gender dysphoria includes three stage treatment:[22]

1) wholly reversible interventions: temporary suspension of pubertal development;[23]
2) partially reversible interventions: administration of masculinising/ feminising hormones; and
3) partially irreversible interventions: reassignment surgery.[24]

I will discuss first the wholly reversible interventions; later in this chapter I will focus on the other two.[25]

8   WHOLLY REVERSIBLE INTERVENTIONS

The first stage of treatment involves the temporary suspension of pubertal development. This is perhaps the most controversial of all medical interventions, and I will explain why. This treatment, where provided, is offered in cases in which gender dysphoria is diagnosed as profound and highly likely to persist. The endogenous production of oestrogen in girls and testosterone in boys is temporarily suppressed. The *gonadotropin-releasing hormone analogues* (GnRHa) are the best available drugs. These act on the pituitary gland and inhibit the pituitary hormone secretion.[26] These drugs are sometimes called 'blockers'. These could be given to children after the onset of puberty, but before the substantial development of secondary sex characteristics. This is around what is known as Tanner Stage 2. Box 5.1 contains a description of the Tanner Stages.[27]

Box 5.1   Tanner Stage

PUBIC HAIR (BOTH MALE AND FEMALE)

Tanner I: no pubic hair at all (typically age ten and under)

Tanner II: small amount of long, downy hair with slight pigmentation at the base of the penis and scrotum (males) or on the labia majora (females) (ten to eleven)

Tanner III: hair becomes more coarse and curly, and begins to extend laterally (twelve to fourteen)

Tanner IV: adultlike hair quality, extending across pubis but sparing medial thighs (thirteen to fifteen)

Tanner V: hair extends to medial surface of the thighs (sixteen plus)

GENITALS (MALE)

Tanner I: prepubertal (testicular volume less than 1.5 ml; small penis of 3 cm or less)

Tanner II: testicular volume between 1.6 and 6 ml; skin on scrotum thins, reddens, and enlarges; penis length unchanged

Tanner III: testicular volume between 6 and 12 ml, scrotum enlarges further, penis begins to lengthen to about 6 cm

Tanner IV: testicular volume between 12 and 20 ml, scrotum enlarges further and darkens, penis increases in length to 10 cm and circumference

Tanner V: testicular volume greater than 20 ml, adult scrotum and penis of 15 cm in length

BREASTS (FEMALE)

Tanner I: no glandular tissue; areola follows the skin contours of the chest (prepubertal)

Tanner II: breast bud forms, with small area of surrounding glandular tissue; areola begins to widen

Tanner III: breast begins to become more elevated and extends beyond the borders of the areola, which continues to widen but remains in contour with surrounding breast

Tanner IV: increased breast size and elevation; areola and papilla form a secondary mound projecting from the contour of the surrounding breast

Tanner V: breast reaches final adult size; areola returns to contour of the surrounding breast, with a projecting central papilla

During the first and second stage of treatment, the child may be encouraged to have what is sometimes called a Real Life Experience.[28] This involves adopting the role of the other gender in order to experience the congruence with presumed innate gender identity. The child, during this process, should also receive psychological support. After experiencing what life is like in the other gender, the child/adolescent might decide to go on with therapy and, eventually, to begin cross sex hormones (see Section 10). Alternatively, s/he might wish to revert to the phenotypical sex and interrupt therapy. By resuming endogenous sex hormone production, the pubertal development is thought to restart as normal. For this reason, 'blockers' are regarded as a *reversible intervention*.

Both the British Society of Paediatric Endocrinology and Diabetes (BSPED)[29] and the Royal College of Psychiatrists in the UK regard puberty suppressant drugs as a *therapeutic tool*. However, they can also be regarded as a *diagnostic tool*, as one of their most important functions is to enhance understanding of the real nature, degree, and persistency of the child's discomfort.[30] Delemarre-van de Waal and Cohen-Kettenis write:

> Making a balanced decision on SR [sex reassignment] is far more difficult for adolescents, who are denied medical treatment (GnRHa included), because much of their energy will be absorbed by obtaining treatment rather than exploring in an open way whether SR actually is the treatment of choice for their gender problem. By starting with GnRHa their motivation for such exploration enhances and no irreversible changes have taken place if, as a result of the psychotherapeutic interventions, they would decide that SR is not what they need.[31]

8.1 At What Stage Should Puberty Be Suspended?

The time at which suppression or inhibition of endogenous sex hormones should begin is controversial. The WPATH's *Standards of Care* (formerly known as the *Harry Benjamin International Gender Dysphoria Association's Standards of Care for Gender Identity Disorders*) states that the minor can receive the hormone blocking medication, provided that s/he has commenced puberty and has had a persistent desire to change sex throughout the childhood.[32] Box 5.2 cites extracts of these guidelines.

Box 5.2   WPATH Standards of Care[33]

Adolescents may be eligible for puberty suppressing hormones as soon as pubertal changes have begun. In order for adolescents and their parents to make an informed decision about pubertal delay, it is recommended that adolescents experience the onset of puberty to at least Tanner Stage 2. Some children may arrive at this stage at very young ages (e.g., 9 years of age. Studies evaluating this approach only included children who were at least 12 years of age [. . .]

Puberty suppression may continue for a few years, at which time a decision is made to either discontinue all hormone therapy or transition to a feminizing/masculinizing hormone regimen. Pubertal suppression does not inevitably lead to social transition or to sex reassignment [. . .]

In order for adolescents to receive puberty suppressing hormones, the following minimum criteria must be met:

1. The adolescent has demonstrated a long-lasting and intense pattern of gender nonconformity or gender dysphoria (whether suppressed or expressed);
2. Gender dysphoria emerged or worsened with the onset of puberty;
3. Any co-existing psychological, medical, or social problems that could interfere with treatment (e.g., that may compromise adherence) have been addressed, such that the adolescent's situation and functioning are stable enough to start treatment;
4. The adolescent has given informed consent and, particularly when the adolescent has not reached the age of medical consent, the parents or other caretakers or guardians have consented to the treatment and are involved in supporting the adolescent throughout the treatment process.[34]

These guidelines offer extensive advice regarding the overall care for minors and adults with atypical gender development. They also stress that before any physical interventions are considered for minors, "extensive exploration of psychological, family, and social issues should be undertaken [. . .]. The duration of this exploration may vary considerably depending on the complexity of the situation".[35]

Importantly, these guidelines are upfront on the goals that the WPATH has. "The overall goal of the SOC [*Standards of Care*] is to provide clinical guidance for health professionals to assist transsexual, transgender, and gender nonconforming people with safe and effective pathways to achieving lasting personal comfort with their gendered selves, in order to maximise their overall hath, psychological well-being, and self-fulfilment".[36] Treatment should be available "to assist people with such distress to explore their gender identity and find a gender role that is comfortable for them". Moreover, "treatment is individualized: what helps one person alleviate gender dysphoria might be very different from what helps another person. This process may or may not involve a change in gender expression or body modifications [. . .]

Gender identities and expressions are diverse, and hormones and surgery are just two of many options available to assist people with achieving comfort with self and identity".[37] The idea is that therapy should not aim at leading the sufferer back to the gender assigned at birth, but instead at helping the individual to understand his or her gender identity and live in it, whatever that may be, and at assisting him or her in this process with a range of interventions, including primary care, psychological support, voice and communication therapy,[38] medical treatment, and surgery when necessary. In other words, the goal should be psychological welfare and social adjustment, and the means to achieve it should be tailored to each individual.

Other recent guidelines for treatment of gender dysphoria have been published in 2009 by the Endocrine Society. The Endocrine Society claims to be:

> The world's oldest, largest, and most active organization devoted to research on hormones and the clinical practice of endocrinology. The Society works to foster a greater understanding of endocrinology amongst the general public and practitioners of complementary medical disciplines and to promote the interests of all endocrinologists at the national scientific research and health policy levels of government.[39]

Box 5.3 reports a summary of the Endocrine Society's recommendations relating to minors. These appear congruent with the WPATH guidelines.

Box 5.3   Endocrine Treatment of Transsexual Persons: An Endocrine Society Clinical Practice Guideline[40]

2.0. TREATMENT OF ADOLESCENTS

2.1. We recommend that adolescents who fulfil eligibility and readiness criteria for gender reassignment initially undergo treatment to suppress pubertal development.

2.2. We recommend that suppression of pubertal hormones start when girls and boys first exhibit physical changes of puberty (confirmed by pubertal levels of estradiol and testosterone, respectively), but no earlier than Tanner stages 2–3.[41]

2.3. We recommend that GnRH analogues be used to achieve suppression of pubertal hormones.

2.4. We suggest that pubertal development of the desired opposite sex be initiated at about the age of 16 years, using a gradually increasing dose schedule of cross-sex steroids.

2.5. We recommend referring hormone-treated adolescents for surgery when 1) the real-life experience (RLE) has resulted in a satisfactory social role change; 2) the individual is satisfied about the hormonal effects; and 3) the individual desires definitive surgical changes.

2.6. We suggest deferring surgery until the individual is at least 18 years old.

These guidelines are completed by a number of recommendations relating to how to follow up and screen patients for possible complications, such as breasts and prostate cancer screening, bone mineral density assessments, and others (I will discuss the issues raised by the Real Life Experience in the next chapter).

The UK Royal College of Psychiatrists, back in 1998, recommended that adolescents have experience of themselves in the postpubertal state of their biological sex. However, it contemplated the possibility of earlier interventions.[42] There are still only very few clinics around the world that deal specifically with minors with gender dysphoria: among these, we should mention Toronto, Boston, New York, Washington, London, Amsterdam, Berlin, Frankfurt, Hamburg, and Havana.[43] Early suspension of puberty is offered in the clinics in Germany, the US, Canada, Australia, the Netherlands, and Belgium.[44] Since 2011, early medical treatment is also offered in London, but within a research study context (see Chapter 7).

However, not everybody agrees with providing medical treatment to minors with gender dysphoria at Tanner Stages 2 or 3. In 2006 BSPED published some guidelines, stating that puberty should be *complete* before any medical treatment could start.[45]

Box 5.4   BSPED[46]

An adolescent should be left to experience his/her natural hormone environment uninterrupted until:
  A) Development of secondary sexual characteristics is complete
  B) Final height has been achieved
  C) Peak bone mass has been accrued (ideally)

Peak bone mass of course accrues at around the age of twenty-five, and therefore in these guidelines medical treatment was in practice denied to minors. BSPED withdrew its approval from its own guidelines in October 2006 after questions were raised about their clinical appropriateness (puberty cannot be 'suspended' if it has already completed its course) and credibility (no date of publication or authorship were claimed). In 2011, the UK Gender Identity Clinic Tavistock and Portman, based in London, released the news that early treatment, including temporary suppression of puberty with administration of GnRHa, can begin within a controlled research study.[47]

However, the opposition to early treatment that the BSPED expressed raised a number of important issues:

1) What sufferers can do if one body of medical opinion holds a practice that somehow diverges from the opinion of *another* body of medical opinion (this will be discussed in Chapter 7).

2) What options people have in countries, such as the UK, where they are entitled to receive publicly funded care, but where their freedom to obtain alternative services, even on a private basis, is limited (this will also be discussed in Chapter 7).
3) What the experience of children who have been treated after completion of pubertal development is: this would help us to understand the ethics of treating transgender minors (this will be discussed here).

The following case history refers to an adolescent who has been provided hormonal treatment *only after completion of puberty.*

CASE HISTORY 1: SIXTEEN-AND-A-HALF-YEAR-OLD (M→F) NOT BEEN TREATED UNTIL PUBERTAL DEVELOPMENT WAS COMPLETE

I [. . .] began my puberty at the age of ten, so I have lived with this profound physical wrongness for over six and a half years. The last two and a half years have been horrendous for me, with my body becoming so disgustingly adult male that I cannot bear it. [. . .] My body will never, ever be as I would like it to be and now, unfortunately, it is really a case of damage limitation. [. . .] At the moment, I am living in a limbo land—my name is [. . .] and I dress in female clothes, but I have facial and body hair, which makes me feel horrible. I am the wrong shape for the clothes that I wear and I have genitalia which is completely alien and upsetting and which protrudes through my clothes [. . .] If I could have started on blockers at Tanner Stage Two (this, for me, was at the age of about twelve) [. . .] I would have been able to avoid the worst physical effects of male puberty; as it is, I am going to have to spend years, and a lot of money, trying to get rid of the many physical male attributes that I could have avoided. [. . .] I still have many years of being covered, from head to toe, with thick, black hair to look forward to.[48]

In 2005 Fenner and Mananzala of FIERCE, in collaboration with Z. Arkles and Dean Spade from the Sylvia Rivera Law Project (SRLP), produced a report in which they describe the condition of children who are denied early medications and are left to develop in the 'wrong' body.[49] For many, obtaining hormonal treatment is a life-or-death matter, and many would go through whatever is necessary to facilitate access to treatment, because growing in the alien body is simply not an option for them.[50] This, for many, means seeking help via nonauthorised sources, such as the Internet or the street, taking hormones at nonregulated dosages, with all the physical, psychological, and social consequences this may have (an extract of the report is available in Chapter 6).

Delemarre-van de Waal and Cohen-Kettenis are pioneers in the study of transgenderism in children. They have observed and treated a number of minors with gender variance. They have systematically recorded a number of clinical data, and they conclude that "the experience of a full biological puberty may seriously interfere with healthy psychological functioning and well being".[51] As we shall also see in Chapter 6, in February 2007 the UK newspaper the *Telegraph* reported the news of a twelve-year-old boy treated for gender dysphoria in Germany. This appears to be one of the youngest transgender children officially treated with medication. Experts claimed on that occasion that treatment was administered in light of the *trauma* that can affect trans children when their body begins to take the shape of the unwanted gender.[52] There seems to be a consensus amongst experts that pubertal development can be all around very harmful to children with gender variance.

In order to understand whether there is any sound ethical or clinical reason to defer treatment, thus leaving children and adolescents to grow in their biological phenotype, it is important to gather a better understanding of the clinical benefits and risks of early medical intervention.

KEY POINTS

- Minors with gender dysphoria can be treated medically.
- Gender dysphoria treatment involves three stages: (1) wholly reversible treatment; (2) partly reversible treatment; (3) irreversible treatment.
- The first stage of treatment involves administration of GnRHa, which temporarily suspends puberty.
- International guidelines advise on starting medical treatment not earlier than Tanner Stage 2 or 3.

---

9 SUSPENSION OF PUBERTY: BENEFITS

Temporary suppression of pubertal development has the following advantages:

1. It immediately reduces the patient's suffering.[53] Kreukels and Cohen-Kettenis explain that even trans children who have functioned reasonably well during childhood are usually extremely distressed by the first signs of puberty, and entering puberty may cause them anxiety and depression. "Therefore," they warn, "the suppression of puberty, followed by cross sex hormone treatment and surgery seems to have undeniable benefits for transsexual youths".[54]
2. Suspension of puberty improves the precision of the diagnosis. Adolescents are given more time to explore their self and their gender, without the distress of the changing body.[55]

3. Suspension of puberty can also help identifying children who are false positives. Delemarre-van de Waal and Cohen-Kettenis argue that early administration of blockers might *increase* the incidence of false positives. However, later discussion in their paper suggests that appropriate diagnosis *decreases* the chance of treating false positives.[56]

4. Suspension of puberty reduces the invasiveness of future surgery. In female to male, it would avoid, for example, breast removal; in male to female it would avoid painful and expensive treatment for facial and body hair; moreover, the voice will not deepen, and nose, jaw, and cricoid cartilage (Adam's apple) will be less developed. This will avoid later thyroid chondroplasty to improve appearance and crico-thyroid approximation to raise the pitch of the voice.[57]

5. Better psychosocial adaptation appears associated with early physical intervention.[58] A later review confirmed that "early intervention not only seemed to lead to a better psychological outcome, but also to a physical appearance that made being accepted as a member of the new gender much easier, compared with those who began treatment in adulthood".[59]

10 SUSPENSION OF PUBERTY: RISKS

A major concern is the impact of GnRHa on development. GnRHa has been used for some time in the treatment of prostate cancer patients. Prostate cancer is associated with testosterone production, and inhibition of testosterone reduces the diffusion of cancerous cells. However, when used in the population of transgender children, GnHRa is used somewhat experimentally. I will discuss the ethical and legal issues that this may raise in Chapters 6 and 7. GnRHa is thought to be the most effective medication able to temporarily suspend the development of secondary sex characteristics. Administration of GnRHa slows the pubertal growth spurt. This can represent an advantage for male to female children, as it makes it more likely for them to achieve an ultimate height within the normal female range. However, the obvious question is whether reduction of the rate of growth has any side effects on bone formation and metabolism.[60] GnRHa inhibits the production of endogenous sex hormones and thereby impacts on the formation of bone mass. Later administration of cross sex hormones can increase bone mass, but long term effects on bone mass development and sitting height are unclear. Peak bone mass can only be measured when patients are about twenty-five years old, and such a long term follow up has not yet been performed.

Another concern is the effect of GnRHa on the brain. Males and females show different brain development, especially in amount of grey matter. The effects of suppression of puberty on the brain need to be evaluated.[61]

Currently, the only centres that monitor the consequences of puberty suppressant drugs over an extended period of time are the Departments of Medical Psychology and Pediatrics in Amsterdam. The Amsterdam team see around seventy new children every year. According to their estimates, two-thirds of the *adolescents* (age twelve to eighteen) who apply for treatment are diagnosed as having profound and persistent Gender Identity Disorder and will then be treated. Twenty to twenty-five per cent of *children* (under twelve) who are seen at their centre suffer persisting dysphoria and, following the department's procedures of assessment, will be treated once they reach puberty.[62]

These estimates should only be taken as a rough indication. Given that patients who are refused therapy or who decide to suspend therapy are not followed up, it is impossible to establish whether they will eventually transition to the other gender as adults, whether they will adjust to one gender or not, or whether they will seek medical care elsewhere. This might be inevitable, but to some extent impinges upon the reliability of statistics of incidence and prevalence of transgenderism in the general population and on the way atypical gender develops when it is manifested early in life (for more on incidence and prevalence, see Chapter 4).

The selection process in Amsterdam includes strict psychological and endocrinological assessments. Until they undergo surgery (after the age of eighteen) patients are seen by the endocrinologist and by the psychologist at least every three months, although the psychologist is available for more frequent sessions. The endocrinological and psychological follow up is meant to observe and prevent any abnormal development and adverse consequences of treatment. All parties should be convinced that treatment is in the best interests of the child.[63]

Follow up includes assessment of bone density and body composition— yearly; skeletal age—yearly; endocrine and metabolic parameters—every six months; and anthropometry (overall height, weight, sitting height, skin folds, waist and hips)—every three months. "Laboratory measurements include levels of gonadotropins and sex hormones, metabolic parameters such as fasting glucose, insulin, cholesterol, high-density lipoprotein and low-density lipoprotein levels. In addition, safety parameters, such as renal and liver functions, are estimated".[64]

These studies show that later administration of cross sex hormones makes it possible to manipulate overall height and achieve *quasi* normal height.[65]

Additional concerns regarding blockers are their effects on reproductive capability. Specialists in Belgium have explored these effects.[66] De Sutter explains that the use of blockers in early puberty might prevent the storage of sperm (for male to female children) and of ova (for female to male children) for future reproductive purposes. However, the suppression of spermatogenesis in males is temporary and can be restored by interrupting treatment. A boy whose puberty has been suppressed before spermatogenesis has occurred could decide to stop treatment long enough for spermatogenesis to start, once he is a bit older, if he wishes to collect and store sperm for reproductive purposes (this of course would mean that he would have to accept the masculinising effects of endogenous testosterone on his body). He can then continue with treatment for transition to female gender.

Collection of ova in females is less problematic. The treatment has little impact on the already formed ova. They may be collected and stored at the time of oophorectomy.[67]

An additional problem for trans girls is that the genital tissue available for the later creation of a vagina will be less than would otherwise have been available, but this problem could be resolved with appropriate surgical intervention.[68]

The results of current studies are encouraging. Suspension of puberty at an early stage seems to have no significant and uncontrollable adverse side effects. Peter Lee and Christopher Houk write: "We believe suppression of pubertal sexual characteristics is warranted when there is evidence of pubertal onset. Suppression of pubertal sex steroid production and thus secondary sexual characteristics can be effectively and safely accomplished using gonadotropin-releasing hormone analogues (GnRHa)—an intervention that is both temporary and reversible".[69]

Normal Spack, an endocrinologist at Harvard, reports that, of seventy adolescents he had in care, one-third had suicidal ideation and 10 per cent attempted suicide. After hormonal treatment was prescribed, none of these children had suicidal ideation.[70] Therefore, medication seems to have a decisively beneficial impact on distress.

Preliminary evidence leads to the conclusion that there are sound clinical grounds for commencing treatment soon after the onset of puberty. Questions can be raised, however, as to the *ethical* legitimacy of suspension of puberty. These will be discussed Chapter 6. I shall now move to those interventions that are only partially reversible, those that, once provided, produce changes that can no longer be altered or that can only be altered with medical or surgical procedures.

11 PARTIALLY REVERSIBLE INTERVENTIONS

Partially reversible interventions refer to masculinising and feminising hormones.

Cross sex hormones have the following benefits:

1. They initiate the development of the secondary sex characteristics that accord with the perceived gender identity (for female to male patients, deepened voice, clitoral enlargement, growth of facial and body hair, cessation of menses, atrophy of breast tissue, increased libido, decreased percentage of body fat compared to muscle mass; in

male to female patients, breast growth, decreased libido and testicular size, increased percentage of body fat compared to muscle mass).[71]
2. They make it easier for the person to have a Real Life Experience by beginning to alter the physical appearance to accord with the new gender role.
3. They allow the person to explore what it feels like to be the other gender, thus making it possible to make a better informed choice about irreversible interventions.

The correct administration of masculinising/feminising hormones is a crucial issue in treatment of minors with gender dysphoria.[72] The case history that follows illustrates how disagreement in protocols may affect the patient's welfare.

CASE HISTORY 2: DIFFERENCES IN ADMINISTRATION OF MASCULINISING/FEMINISING HORMONES

A sixteen-and-a-half-year-old (male to female) at Tanner Stage 5 (and therefore already fully grown in the biological male phenotype) is treated in the UK with analogue GnHRa, followed later by 5 mcg of ethinylestradiol per day. This would be increased every six months. In Gent, in Amsterdam, and in the US, ethinylestradiol is not utilised in cases like hers. Beta estradiol (in the US this is called Estrace) is used, because it is a natural oestrogen and because it has shown lower association with thrombosis. The dosage of beta estradiol that she would be recommended is comparable to 30–50 mcg of ethinylestradiol— much higher than the dosage the patient had received in the UK. The patient in this case reports dissatisfaction, and her views are persistently dismissed, until she manages to obtain private treatment travelling to the US. Full satisfaction follows the new treatment protocol.[73]

The difference in national protocols has the inevitable and unfortunate consequence of promoting 'medical tourism'. US experts report that patients who are not treated adequately in some European countries travel to the US to receive privately paid treatment.[74] Those who cannot afford this are forced to suffer or attempt other, often illegal, and, more importantly, unsafe routes, as we saw in the preceding.

Thus, perhaps, one further 'benefit' could be added to the list: prevention of entanglement with unsafe sources of medication and possibly hazardous lifestyles. Whether this benefit, which is not strictly speaking a *clinical* benefit, should be of concern to doctors and should be ethically relevant in decisions as to whether these medications should be provided will be discussed in Chapters 6 and 7.

12   RISKS ASSOCIATED WITH CROSS SEX HORMONES

The WPATH *Standards of Care* reads that "To date, no controlled clinical trials of any feminizing/masculinizing hormone regimen have been conducted to evaluate safety or efficacy in producing physical transition. As a result, wide variation in doses and types of hormones have been published in the medical literature [. . .]"[75]. However, a broad overview of the risks associated with cross sex hormones may be found in literature.

Risks of cross sex hormones are mainly cardiovascular. Cross sex hormones seem to increase the likelihood of occurrence of serious/fatal cardiovascular diseases in patients already at risk (smokers, obese patients, patients with heart diseases, hypertension, clotting abnormalities, or some endocrine abnormalities). Most of these risks concern mainly adults and generally do not apply to children and adolescents with gender dysphoria.

In trans women, estrogens and progestin may cause infertility, weight gain, emotional lability, liver disease, gallstone formation, somnolence, and diabetes mellitus. In trans men, testosterone may cause infertility, acne, emotional lability, increased sexual desire, hepatic dysfunction, and even malignant liver tumours.[76] In 1991 the *Lancet* warned about increased cancer morbidity and mortality relating to intake of hormones in transsexual patients.[77]

One final important risk associated with cross sex hormones is that the treatment is only partially reversible. If a patient decides to interrupt treatment, effects such as voice change and beard growth cannot be changed, although possibly ameliorated, and breast development in males through administration of estrogens and progestin can be only removed with surgery.[78]

The WPATH guidelines suggest that "adolescents may be eligible to begin feminising/masculinising hormone therapy, preferably with parental consent. In many countries, 16-year-olds are legal adults for medical decision-making and do not require parental consent. Ideally, treatment decisions should be made among the adolescent, the family, and the treatment team".[79] I will examine the ethical and legal issues around the involvement of the family in Chapters 6 and 7.

13   IRREVERSIBLE INTERVENTIONS

Surgery represents the final stage of treatment, although hormone intervention may be an additional lifelong treatment. The benefits of surgery are evident. The patient has finally obtained a body in line with the innate gender identity. Some report the experience as a 'rebirth'. For example, Vladimir Luxuria, in her book *The Unspoken Tales*, narrates in a literary style the transition of a male to female as follows:

He woke up slowly, and saw his father holding his hand. . . 'Don't worry, it's over now. . .', he said to her. But she felt stoned, she was bandaged and felt a strange sensation between her legs, and also all the rubber tubes hanging from her arms, like the yarns of a marionette [. . .]. He feared moving, and unplugging all those rubber tubes [. . .]. The doctor explained: 'When the effect of painkillers fades out, you will start feeling pain. Do not worry, this is normal. When you can't bear them, then push this button and a nurse will come immediately to give you more painkillers [. . .]. From now onwards you won't be Claudio any more. We shall call you with the name with which you have decided to be born again [. . .] The intervention has been easy, all has gone well. Now you will have to cope with the normal postoperative rehabilitation. We are proud of ourselves and happy for you. You have decided that your name will be Luce, and for us you will always be our Luce'.[80]

According to a study, body satisfaction significantly increases in the vast majority of cases after medical treatment and surgery.

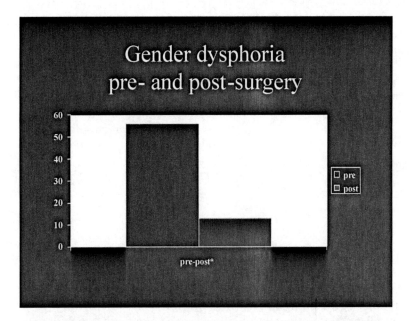

Figure 5.1 Clinical management of adolescents with gender dysphoria.

Source: Peggy T. Cohen-Kettenis and Henriette Delemarre-van de Waal, Departments of Medical Psychology and Pediatrics, VU Medical Center, Amsterdam, the Netherlands.[81]

Risks of surgery include normal risks associated with all surgery.[82] Specific risks for male to female patients include "complete or partial necrosis of the vagina and labia, fistulas from the bladder or bowel into the vagina, stenosis of the urethra,[83] and vaginas that are too small or short for coitus".[84] There are specific risks associated to female to male surgery: "metoidioplasty results in micropenis, without the capacity for standing urination. Phalloplasty [. . .] is a lengthy, multi-stage procedure with significant morbidity that includes frequent urinary complications and unavoidable donor site scarring".[85]

Additional risks concern body dissatisfaction,[86] albeit cases in which the person wishes to revert to the original gender are rare.[87] Still relatively rare, as the study from Cohen-Kettenis and Delemarre-van de Waal shows, is incomplete satisfaction. In these cases, the reasons for partial satisfaction can be diverse. For example, it may be hard for female to male transgenders to obtain metaidoioplasty or phalloplasty.[88] In the Netherlands, for example, there is a long waiting list, and in other countries this surgery is not provided by the national healthcare system. This could be an important reason for body dissatisfaction.[89] Incomplete satisfaction might be a function of the life history of those who transition. It is possible that many of those who have had to struggle a great deal to obtain medical care experience significant uncertainty over the sense of self due to their life experiences. Or, in other cases, partial satisfaction may be due to the fact that being 'one or the other' is not the solution to all forms of gender dysphoria: not everyone adapts themselves to the rigid gender divide.

International guidelines advise that surgery should not be carried out before the age of eighteen, or before the age of majority in a given country.[90] In September 2007 the courts of Argentina granted permission for cross sex surgery to a seventeen-year-old patient, Natalia.[91]

14 CONCLUSION

Gender dysphoria is associated with great distress and poor psychosocial outcome, especially in cases in which proper intervention is not offered efficiently and in a timely manner. This chapter has discussed what types of approaches have historically been used with children and adolescents with gender variance, their theoretical underpinnings, and their goals. As I noted before, there is consensus that a combined approach is the most promising, and various international guidelines provide advice as to how to organise it.

This chapter has also assessed the risks and benefits of the medical treatments available. No medical intervention is risk free. Indeed, no human activity is risk free. And, indeed, perhaps no human *omission* is risk free either. One needs to accept that a risk free choice is probably not a given.

Yet, the fact that there are potential risks associated with the administration of treatment to minors has given rise to much concern about the morality and lawfulness of these therapies. In the next chapter, I will discuss the major ethical issues associated with treatment for gender dysphoria in minors. I will focus in particular on the first stage of treatment, because this is the most controversial amongst all treatments for gender dysphoria, and because it gives rise to profound ethical dilemmas, which need to be disentangled for the benefit of both treating clinicians and their younger patients.

KEY POINTS

- Gender dysphoria in minors can be treated medically.
- International guidelines advise suspension of puberty with GnRHa.
- Suspension of puberty is offered in several countries.
- Suspension of puberty is wholly reversible.
- Analysis of risks/benefits shows that GnRHa is a benign drug.
- No uncontrollable side effects are shown in clinical studies.
- Partly reversible interventions include masculinising/feminising hormones.
- Irreversible interventions include various surgical treatments.
- Body dissatisfaction after surgery is rare.
- International guidelines advise that surgery should only be offered to adults.

6 Ethical Issues Surrounding Treatment of Transgender Minors

Inside this Good, and inside this Evil, I feel estranged. I am a foreigner of Morality.

(Jacques Brel)[1]

1 INTRODUCTION

Transgenderism is often described as a sense of 'estrangement' (see Chapter 4). I have in the course of the book referred to transgenders as a *minority*, which also connects with the description of transgenderism as a sense of 'estrangement'; I have also linked transgenderism to anarchy, to the refusal of authority, implying that a rigid classification of genders is an authority that does not represent all the people. The study of transgenderism thus is in one important sense the study (somewhat political) of the way majorities deal with minorities. But in another sense the study of transgenderism requires some introspection and challenges us to reconsider what is normal for a human being and what is not, what is ordinary and what is atypical, what is healthy and what is pathological, what should be corrected and what should be respected. Transgenderism thus challenges us to reconsider us all as being beyond the boundaries, as it is those very boundaries that fade as one tries to understand transgenderism. Dealing with transgenderism, thus, in one important way, inevitably challenges us to rethink good and bad, right and wrong, and to become, thus, *foreigners of Morality*.

In this chapter, I focus on the ethical issues arising in connection with the medical treatment for children with gender dysphoria. This does not, of course, exhaust all the ethical predicaments that rotate around the treatment and care of these children. However, the main ethical objections to such treatment will be considered.

2 THE TREATMENT OF TRANSGENDER CHILDREN

A boy of 12 is believed to have become the world's youngest sex change patient after convincing doctors that he wanted to live the rest of his life as a female. . . . The therapy involves artificially arresting male puberty, with a series of potent hormone injections. (Telegraph)[2]

The treatment of children and adolescents belonging to the gender minority is abundant in ethical problems. One important conceptual and ethical issue is whether gender variance is appropriately regarded as a mental illness. Chapter 8 will discuss this point. Several researchers have argued that the inclusion of Gender Identity Disorder (GID) in the DSM and other diagnostic manuals is unjustifiable or at least dubious (see Chapter 8). But there are many other ethical and legal issues specifically concerning the treatment of children and adolescents.

In the previous chapter, we have seen that children and adolescents can be treated with hormonal medications as early as Tanner Stage 2 or 3. At the beginning of puberty, their pubertal development can be temporarily arrested. If it were possible to predict which children will be persisters, it would even be possible to initiate medical treatment earlier, before the onset of puberty (see Chapter 5). Currently, the reaction of the child to pubertal development is used diagnostically. This is, of course, risky, as it means subjecting the child to potentially avoidable trauma, and it also means exposing the child to future mutilating surgery, which could be prevented.

Medical treatment for children, which involves the administration of puberty suppressant drugs, has been at the centre of animated debates internationally. In several clinics around the world this treatment is offered. In the UK, however, there has been strong resistance to initiate treatment before puberty is complete, and only in 2011 did UK specialists decide to provide such treatment earlier, within a carefully monitored research study.[3]

The main arguments against providing treatment to children with gender variance are:

- This is playing god.
- This is a social problem, not a medical problem.
- Experimental treatment is unethical.
- Children with gender dysphoria are not competent to make these types of decisions. Discussing this argument involves clarifications on the law relating to treatment of minors with so called 'mental illnesses', and I will consider this in the next chapter.

3   PLAYING GOD

One of the main issues that can be raised about early medical treatment is that this is *like playing god* or *playing with nature*. There might be an intuitive distrust or revulsion to medical interventions that interfere with spontaneous development. Fiddling with puberty, using medications to interfere with the natural development of a child at such a delicate stage of growth, may seem morally unacceptable. However, it is not clear why human life should not be interfered with, when the purpose of the interference is to alleviate suffering or ameliorate people's lives. Many contemporary philosophers have made this important point.⁴ But even in the history of philosophy earlier thinkers insisted on the idea that an appeal to nature does not say much about what is good or right. In Chapter 2, when discussing the notion of gender, we saw that John Stuart Mill made a similar consideration on the role of women in society: one cannot ethically appeal to 'nature' to justify how people are treated. In an essay on suicide, David Hume made a similar point. Hume published his essay in 1783. There was no law at the time in Scotland on suicide, but in England and in other parts of the world suicide was a crime under the law, and it was considered (as it is today by some religions) as against god's will and as a capital sin. Hume defended people's moral right to take their lives and argued that such an act cannot justifiably be regarded as a sin or as against god's will or as against nature. While considering this last point (that suicide is immoral because it is against 'nature', it is 'playing god'), Hume wrote the following passage, which is still relevant to us today for its cogent insight and lucid analysis.

> Were the disposal of human life so much reserved as the peculiar province of the Almighty. . . it would be equally criminal to act for the preservation of life. . . If I turn aside a stone which is falling upon my head, I disturb the course of nature, and I invade the peculiar province of the Almighty, by lengthening out my life beyond the period which by the general laws of matter and motion he had assigned it. . . any why not impious, say I, to build houses, cultivate the ground, or sail upon the ocean? In all these actions we employ our powers of mind and body, to produce some innovation in the course of nature; and in none of them do we any more.⁵

Medicine is a discipline aimed at changing the course of events and nature, hopefully for the better.⁶ All medicine is an interference with nature; pain in labour, for example, is a normal and spontaneous part of a *natural event*. Yet pain relief is neither unethical nor unlawful *just because* it is an interference with nature. Ageing carries adverse effects for our health, and it is a known fact that this is a process that goes with human nature; yet it is neither morally nor legally wrong to interfere with this process of spontaneous development in order to ameliorate people's quality of life. Interfering with spontaneous developments, if they cause harm, is not only ethically legitimate, but also *good*: it promotes happiness, it makes people's lives better, and it minimises suffering. Insofar as interference with what is thought of as a 'spontaneous' development is likely to achieve these aims, there is a strong *prima facie* moral reason in favour of interfering. Of course, if it is right to intervene to delay ageing at one end of spontaneous development, it should be right to delay ageing at the other end for the same purposes. Thus, there is no reason to believe that interfering with nature, or with development, is inherently a bad thing, and this objection does not provide a sound ground for denying treatment that could be beneficial.

4   THIS IS A SOCIAL PROBLEM, NOT A MEDICAL PROBLEM

The idea that transsexualism is a social problem, and therefore should not be medicalised, is one that has run through literature. The literature has traditionally dealt principally with adults, but the point is one of relevance in the case of children as well.

As early as 1979 Jon Meyer at the Johns Hopkins Medical Institution proposed a similar argument. Meyer argued that surgery (although his argument can be extended to other medical interventions) is not useful in the resolution of the problems of transgenders, because their problems are psychiatric in nature, and physical interventions cannot resolve those psychiatric problems.[7] In Chapter 8 I will discuss whether there are sound epistemological reasons to consider gender variance as a psychiatric or a psychological disorder, and I will conclude that such reasons are lacking. We have also seen in Chapter 5 that purely psychological treatment has poor outcomes. It should also be noted that medical and pharmacological treatment is routinely used to treat the so called 'symptoms' of many so called 'psychiatric disorders'. It is not clear why, even if transsexualism was a psychiatric disorder (and I will argue that it is not), transsexuals should not be treated in the same way as other 'psychiatric' patients.

Another objection raised against medical treatment for transgenderism is that gender variance is a psychological response to a perhaps 'disordered' society, which imposes strong gender stereotypes. The sufferer is lacerated by social demands that s/he cannot satisfy, in that s/he cannot conform to the expected roles. A masculine femininity and a feminine masculinity are not foreseen in the sociocultural context of many Western countries, and this is why, according to this argument, non-conforming individuals end up seeking medical treatment, when they could in principle live their gender liminalities undisturbed. It is society that needs to change: society must be prepared to accept the expression of various masculinities and femininities, and people should not bend and mould their bodies; they should not give in to the oppression that creates transsexualism in the first place. By changing people's bodies, rather than social expectations, a twofold harm results: a mutilation of individuals, who are exposed to the risks and pains of extensive surgery, and a reinforcement of the oppressive stereotypes that are at the heart of their suffering.

Raymond has been adamant on this basis to argue that gender dissatisfaction cannot and should not be dealt with by medical means. She writes:

> When used in conjunction with other words such as *gender dissatisfaction, gender discomfort,* or *gender dysphoria,* it [gender] conveys that these can only be altered by very specialized therapy and/or sophisticated technical means. Feminists have described *gender dissatisfaction* in very different terms—i.e., as *sex-role oppression, sexism,* etc. It is significant that there is no specialized or therapeutic vocabulary of *black dissatisfaction, black discomfort* or *black dysphoria* that has been institutionalized in black identity clinics. Likewise, it would be

rather difficult and somewhat humorous to talk about *sex-role oppression clinics*. What the word *gender* ultimately achieves is a classification of sex-role oppression as a therapeutic problem, amenable to therapeutic solutions.[8] (emphasis in the original)

She continues by arguing that "transsexualism is basically a social problem whose cause cannot be explained except in relation to the sex roles and identities that a patriarchal society generates".[9]

Raymond goes as far as to compare medical treatment for gender dysphoria to "rape, sexual abuse, wife-beating, and violent crimes".[10] She argues that these practices, like medical treatment for gender dysphoria, spring from the same patriarchal model of what is 'appropriate' behaviour for women. Not coincidentally, the healthcare profession treating trans people is populated by men: even trans women are *made by men*. Trans surgery is thus a form of sexual politics, and the stress on the social dimension of the problem leads Raymond to the following conclusions: towards the end of her work, medical treatment for gender dysphoria is compared to the Nazi's 'medical' practices, and in some ways presented as even worse than that, in that the trans has so strongly internalised the gender stereotypes that he or she is not openly forced, but has become willing to seek and consent to the mutilating procedures.[11] The transsexual is thus a masochist: "Transsexuals, as masochists, have great difficulty in believing in the validity and sanctity of their own insides. They are attempting to gain a sense of self not only through the acquisition of a new body, but through the pain involved in this process. Physical pain is a constant reminder to transsexuals that they are finally coming alive".[12]

It has been argued in Chapters 2 and 3 that gender identity is a complex product of biological and social forces, as well as individual interpretations. This is true of *all* gender identities, those of the majorities and those of the minorities. In spite of the important contribution of biology to gender development, it appears that a significant proportion of the suffering in gender minorities is caused by social factors. In light of these, one could indeed argue that it is unethical to provide medical treatment. It is unethical to use medicine to resolve a social problem. If 'Gender Identity Disorder' is caused by mistaken social stereotypes, by a rigid gender divide, by prejudice against gender minorities, then these are the variables that need to be tackled. Stereotypes should be amended, and we shouldn't mutilate people's bodies instead. This, in itself, appears a sound argument with a laudable purpose, but at further scrutiny it is untenable.

4.1   Responses

At the end of the day, reasonableness and authentic social life are found more in that emarginated and humiliated part of our society than amongst the powerful.[13]

The hypothesis that when the gender dysphoric seeks medical alteration of their appearance to become physically similar to the person of the opposite sex, they are embracing the very gender stereotypes that are responsible for their discomfort is at least incomplete. Raymond writes:

> Through hormonal and surgical means, transsexuals reject their 'native' bodies, especially their sexual organs, in favour of the body and the sexual organs of the opposite sex. They do this mainly because the body and the genitalia, especially, come to incarnate the essence of their rejected masculinity and desired femininity. Thus transsexualism is the result of socially prescribed definitions of masculinity and femininity, one of which the transsexual rejects in order to gravitate toward the other.[14]

First, this is false. Many transsexuals do not transition fully: many trans women seek breast implants and leave their genitals as they are. Many live in the other gender without any surgery, and many embrace different segments of genders in their identity. It is the discomfort with the body and the roles that the body may incarnate that lead to challenge the entire lifestyle, not only the genitals. What Raymond says offers an implausible interpretation based on what probably a small section of gender dysphoric people chooses to do, namely, full genital transition. By not accounting for the variety of gender expressions that is found in the trans community and indeed in humankind as a whole, the conclusion offered is thus methodologically flawed and unsubstantiated.

Second, providing medical treatment to gender minorities is not responding with medicine to a problem that is social in nature. This is responding with medicine to a serious condition that causes enormous distress to the sufferers and makes them prefer unqualified medical help, street life, and even death to a life in an alien body. Paradoxically, for Raymond the fact that many transsexuals end up resorting to prostitution is an indication of how the transsexual woman has internalised social ideals of femininity: the transsexual accepts the "sexual objectification—prostitution becomes related to the new feminine status"[15] (specifically in the case of male to female transsexuals). Apart from the obvious question as to how we should then explain prostitution for the female to male transsexual (in an interesting report, a female to male transsexual openly discusses how since he has transitioned he can more freely enjoy casual sex just for the sake of it: "I don't want to get up the next morning and have breakfast with this person. I don't want to know his name or phone number. I just want sex. In the women's community, this kind of sexual expression is almost unheard of"[16]), a more important flaw emerges from this argument, one that trivialises and overlooks the important social causes for the drama of prostitution and street life, which indeed affects many belonging to the gender minority. Raymond herself recognises that "frequently they [transsexuals] cannot get jobs [. . .]; the street becomes the breadwinner and the principal place of social contact".[17] For clandestine immigrants, the street is the obvious, and perhaps sometimes the only, place to turn to raise money for privately paid medical treatment. But, similarly, citizens who are either turned down at clinics or who face employment discrimination as transsexual applicants, find an obvious source of income on the pavement. And, of course, they find better acceptance by their peers. Trans may thus choose street life for valid reasons: it may offer the least of various evils. Fenner et al. identify in the rejection from healthcare services perhaps the main factor precipitating gender minorities into street life.

> First, it [being rejected at clinics. . .] alienates [sufferers] from medical providers [. . .]. Because of this increased distrust, many may not return for primary care, HIV testing, STD treatment and other essential care [. . .] These denials also create a necessity [. . .] to seek this care out elsewhere. For many, this care is the only way to express their gender fully so that they can seek employment, attend school, and deal with every day interactions in their new gender. Without hormones, many have a difficult time being perceived by others correctly, opening them up to consistent harassment and violence. For many young people [medical treatment] feels like a life or death need, and they will do whatever is necessary to get this treatment. Many, when rejected at a clinic [. . .], buy their hormones from friends or on the street, injecting without medical supervision at dosages that may not be appropriate and without monitoring by medical professionals. This opens them up to high risk for HIV, hepatitis, and other serious health concerns. Additionally, many youth have difficulty raising money to buy these hormones illegally because they do not have parental support for their transition and face severe job discrimination as young transgender applicants. For many, criminalized behaviour such as prostitution is the only way to raise the money. Doing this work makes them vulnerable to violence, trauma, HIV, and STD infection, and entanglement in the [. . .] justice system.[18]

Thus to say that prostitution reveals how the transsexual has accepted the stereotype of femininity, how prostitution relates to "their new feminine status",[19] how it is a symptom of the transsexual's acceptance and dwelling on his or her 'sexual objectification' is at best simplistic and at worse offensive.

Third, the fact (if this could be demonstrated) that a condition is primarily or solely the result of social factors (maybe of morally wrong social factors) in itself does not imply that medical treatment should not or could not be ethically provided. Indeed, the biological contributions to gender development and to gender dysphoria have been discussed in Chapters 3 and 4. But even if there was no identifiable biological trigger to gender dysphoria, this would have no bearing upon the ethics of providing medical assistance. This will be argued at further length in Chapter 9, but it is important here to anticipate some considerations.

There is a complex debate in applied ethics as to what constitutes an illness or a disease.[20] The extent to which various perils are caused by social stereotypes, and what this reveals about people's entitlement to medical care and about the clinical and moral appropriateness of medical care, is not as simple as it is suggested by the argument analysed here (that if a condition is the result of social forces, then medical treatment should not be provided). It is in fact normal clinical practice to offer medical treatment for conditions of suffering that are not caused by physical or biological imbalances and which are purely determined by social variables or norms (even by morally dubious social norms). The treatment of children with so called 'retarded' growth, or 'excessive' growth, is an example of how endocrinology intervenes to treat conditions that involve no somatic dysfunction[21] and whose distress is associated solely with 'expectations' relating to what is 'normal', and not with pain or physical inability or illness. Treatment in these cases is offered purely on psychological grounds, and the 'disorder' is purely caused by social stereotypes of normality.[22] Treatment for bat ears in children, or circumcision in male infants and children (still legal in England), or 'corrective' surgery for some forms of intersex are other examples of invasive medical treatment administered purely for social reasons (for an account of intersex, or DSDs, see Chapter 2).

Similarly, not wanting children is often a matter of social and cultural variables, but this does not make provision of contraceptive advice and treatment unethical.

Treatment to enhance fertility is also provided (and often publicly funded or reimbursed under insurance schemes) even if infertility is not *stricto sensu* an illness: for some people it is indeed an advantaged state (and many seek temporary and permanent infertility treatment), and for others is an indifferent state. Of course, many delay the date of maternity and paternity for social reasons (later age of employability, career requirements, and the like) and have no 'illness': their reduced fertility is a natural function of age, and their need for medical help is a *social product or a social construct*. Lesbians and single women who apply for assisted reproduction often have no underlying pathology and yet need and can obtain medical assistance to procreate.

When fertility treatment is provided to the groups mentioned in the preceding, various factors are taken into account (suitability of the applicant, the interests of any child affected by this potential birth and so on[23]). Why people are infertile or why they are made to suffer by being childless is not an issue. Many women might suffer being childless primarily because they have internalised the idea that, in order to be 'complete', a woman should also be a mother; others might suffer because they disappoint an expectation of their partners or social groups. Whether women suffer for a 'genuinely' autonomous frustrated wish to procreate or for acquired values or perhaps 'mistaken' or 'suspect' social expectations or norms or gender stereotypes is irrelevant to the medical decision (besides being a question that cannot be answered).

It cannot be up to the endocrinologists or surgeons to perform an analysis of the more profound psychological or social reasons some people want children, or suffer being childless, or why they ended up wanting kids so late. Medicine cannot scrutinise whether the desire for maternity is a biological instinct, or rather a social construct, or make pervasive inspections and judgments of people's life choices and provide fertility treatment accordingly. There is no reason to apply different standards to treatment relating to gender identity (unless a morally relevant difference could be found which justifies differences in treatment).

There might be ethical and pragmatic issues of resource allocation, which could explain why the state might not publicly fund some treatments (see Chapter 9). However, these concerns are not principled reasons to deny medical treatment for conditions that are socially constructed in a significant way, which is the argument analysed here.

Of course, this also raises another conceptual issue relating to how 'social problems' can be sensibly differentiated from 'true medical conditions', an issue outlined earlier by means of the examples of 'retarded' or 'excessive' growth, infertility, bat ears, and many others, and whose conceptual complexity can be compared to the temporal quandary of the chicken and the egg.

Finally, there is, of course, the other issue as to why gender minorities should be turned into martyrs of social ideals. Raymond suggests that "there are many ethical objections to alleviating individual gender suffering at the expense of reinforcing, qualitatively and quantitatively, sex-role conformity", [24] and it is ironic that she writes this in the context of contesting the Nazi's experimentations. By suggesting that individuals should bear avoidable suffering because to alleviate their suffering would harm society, she proposes what she reproaches the Nazis for doing: turning individuals into martyrs of the social good. Of course, in principle, nobody should be allowed to suffer if his or her suffering can be alleviated. If this principle had to be abridged it should be only on very stringent grounds and perhaps in exceptional circumstances. Raymond suggests that medicine here contravenes to one of its first imperatives: *primum non nocere*, first do no harm. A principle of nonmaleficence is included in virtually all moral codes. Suggesting that transsexuals should bear with their pains for the sake of society defies the very principle of nonmaleficence, by imposing avoidable harm to an individual for the sake of others (or, better, *for the sake of an opinion*, because Raymond's argument that medical intervention for transgenderism harms others is at least doubtful).[25]

If gender minorities had to be refused medical care because theirs is 'a social and not a medical problem', they would be jeopardised twice: once because they suffer from a social wrong in the first instance, and the second time because they are denied medical care in the name of that society that harmed them.

Thus, in conclusion, there is no room in the ethical discourse for the argument that transsexualism is a social problem and *therefore should not be treated medically*. It is not clear that gender variance is solely the product of gender stereotypes, and even if it were (a claim that cannot be possibly substantiated given the complexities involved in gender development, as outlined earlier in the book), this would not imply that medical treatment should not be offered.

Of course, one may question whether medical treatment is effective if the causes of the illness are social and not biological. But medical treatment for gender dysphoria eases the suffering and improves social and psychological outcomes, both in the short and long term (see Chapter 5), and if many afflicted by the condition continue to seek it, this further illustrates that the gains, for them, outweigh the risks.

One final point should be made regarding the 'sample' of observed subjects. Many studies, be they by feminists or anthropologists,[26] on transsexualism have looked at adults. Then they have at times provided interpretations based on the experiences of adults. This is a recurrent methodological problem in trans literature: from narrations of adults, and of relatively small samples (Raymond claims to have 'interviewed' ten or fifteen trans, but she does not say much more about her methodology), interpretations or conclusions on the condition are drawn. The problem is that what happens to adults (to a small number of adults willing to be interviewed) cannot be understood without an analysis of the process of gender development and without exploring what happens to children. From the narration of an adult transsexual all a scientist can hope to obtain is his or her personal history, and perhaps some insight on his or her experiences: it is a methodological mistake to generalise from individual narrations and provide interpretations and explanations of the condition generally. The interpretation of transsexualism as a social construct rests in part on this methodological mistake. This interpretation does not account for the experience of children, who may be uncomfortable with their gender at a young age, and whose parents often note the presence of a problem (or a peculiarity) very early in the children's life. It is not always the case that parents ostracise the gender expression of a child. A female to male transsexual, for example, narrates: "I was fortunate enough to have a mother who allowed me great latitude to express masculinity, who in fact said nothing when I decided to wear my brother's clip-on tie to kindergarten with my usual cut-off shorts".[27] Of course the notion of *gender* may be internalised by very young children, and if children's 'variant' gender expressions were accepted socially, they would suffer less. But this does not *per se* imply that either gender or transgenderism is socially constructed.

As the World Professional Association for Transgender Health (WPATH) recognises, health depends not only on good clinical care, but also on "social and political climates that provide and ensure social tolerance, equality, and the full rights of citizenship. Health is promoted through public policies and legal reforms that promote tolerance and equity for gender and sexual diversity and that eliminate prejudice, discrimination, and stigma".[28] "Finding a comfortable gender role", the WPATH writes, "is first and foremost a psychosocial process [. . .], the social aspects of the experience are usually challenging—often more so than the physical aspects".[29] But there is no reason to believe that one type of intervention (social) excludes the other (medical).

5 EXPERIMENTAL TREATMENT IN CHILDREN IS UNETHICAL

Part of the treatment for children and adolescents with gender dysphoria is experimental (see also Chapter 5). In particular, the administration of so called 'blockers', which temporarily suspend pubertal development, is to some extent tentative. The impact of GnRHa on bone formation and the effects on the brain, as we saw in Chapter 5, are under scrutiny at the time this book is being written (2011), although there appears to be no particular reason for concern.

As surgery is currently only advised to adults (with some notable exceptions),[30] by 'experimental treatment' *for children and adolescents*, I refer particularly to the GnRHa and other hormonal treatments.

In light of the existing uncertainty relating to the long term effects of hormonal treatment for gender dysphoric children, including pubertal suppressant medications, one may ask whether it is ethical to provide such treatments. We need to understand well what this concern is about.

The claim that experimenting on children is unethical can mean (at least) two things:

- *Argument 1:* No genuine consent can be given to *experimental* treatment, and lack of proper consent impinges upon the ethical legitimacy of that intervention.[31]
- *Argument 2:* Even if the person can give genuine consent, exposing others, especially children, to unknown risks is unethical.

Let us analyse *argument 1* first. This argument would suggest that one of the core features of valid consent to any medical intervention is information. In treatment for gender variance we do not have full information on the risks and benefits of medications (see Chapter 5). Moreover, children and adolescents might be believed to be more at risk of giving invalid consent, as, arguably, they have greater difficulty in foreseeing how they will feel in the future, due to their limited capacity at long term judgment, their more scanty knowledge of their self, and because gender identity may still be fluctuating during adolescence.

These arguments should be questioned. If it were impossible to consent to interventions whose outcome is uncertain, it would follow that medical research involving human beings is always unethical, regardless of whether research participants are children or adults. In order to give valid consent, the applicant or participant must receive as complete information as possible about treatment and has to be informed about the potential risks of each stage of therapy, even if these risks have not been fully established. Patients should be aware that they are able to withdraw their consent to continuation of involvement with the research project or therapy and never be subjected to any inhuman or degrading treatment or avoidable and unwanted harm or injury.[32] Once such information has been provided, the applicant will ponder the potential risks of treatment with its potential benefits, and will set them against all known and actual psychological, social, and physical effects of not receiving treatment. Moreover, the "desire for sex reassignment never arises abruptly in early-onset transsexual adolescents. These individuals and their parents usually report that the wish to have treatment has been present for many years before the actual referral to the clinic".[33]

Argument 2 is no more successful than *argument 1*. *Argument 2* suggests that even if the person has the legal capacity (the notion of legal capacity is discussed in Chapter 7) to take unknown risks, and even if consent is genuine and legally valid, it is still unethical to expose people, especially minors, to unknown side effects that could affect their future. Children, so the argument may go, have limited knowledge of their self and capacity to make long term judgments. Children with gender variance may, in the anxiety of the moment, make choices that they will later regret; their dysphoria may subside spontaneously. There is always time to provide medical treatment, whereas, once it has been provided, the child is subjected to those potential risks, and this could perhaps be avoided.

Although these concerns are understandable, the belief that treatment is unethical if there is a degree of unpredictability is mistaken. It is a mistake with adults and with children, even accepting that a greater degree of caution should be used towards children. The outcome of many medical interventions is never completely known, whether or not they are considered 'experimental'. If the potential risks of a medical treatment were so high and of such a type that no reasonable person would take them, then indeed a question could be raised as to whether it is ethical to offer such a treatment, even if the applicants had full capacity to consent to it and requested it adamantly. However, the evidence collected so far shows that the treatment for children and adolescents with gender dysphoria is not only benign, but also beneficial. GnRHa is reversible and associated with no severe or uncontrollable side effects. Stage 2 treatment has effects that are more difficult to reverse (partially reversible interventions); however, Stage 2 treatment should in principle be administered after Stage 1 treatment and after a careful assessment of how the child reacts to the first phase of treatment (see Chapter 5), and this is an additional reason why Stage 1 treatment is so important: it may prevent the treatment of false positives, of those children who may have some gender dysphoria, but who will not transition.

Current evidence shows that *not being treated* early may be devastating for most children and adolescents with profound and persistent gender dysphoria and that receiving treatment is highly beneficial. The certain and real side effects of *not receiving treatment* might, for many, outweigh the potential risks of this treatment. Informed patients can make a rational choice to take the potential risks of treatment, when the alternative is on balance of probabilities much worse.

It may be worth reporting here another argument against early treatment, which has been produced in the literature. During adolescence, it has been suggested, the ratio of grey to white matter in the prefrontal brain area changes, and there are increases in connectivity between this area and other areas of the brain as well as an increase in dopaminergic activity in prefrontal striatal limbic pathways. These, it is argued, may lead to increased likelihood of making impulsive choices or engaging in risky behaviour. It should, however, be noted that this potential increased predisposition to impulsive choices may lead the young adolescent who does not receive medical care to engage in risky behaviour out of despair. As we have seen, young people who are denied medical care might try to obtain the medications through illegal sources and may even become suicidal. Moreover, as mentioned earlier, the wish to change gender never occurs abruptly, and it is a long term issue for those who eventually are referred to the specialists. It is thus highly unlikely that the wish to undergo treatment for gender dysphoria may be caused by the variations in the central nervous system suggested in the preceding.[34]

If it can reasonably be expected that therapy improves the applicant's quality of life or can save his or her life, it is not unethical to satisfy the request for treatment—it might indeed be unethical to deny treatment. It is unethical to deny what is for many the only possibility of cure.

This has wider clinical and ethical implications. In judging whether or not to treat, healthcare professionals should evaluate *what is likely to happen to the applicant if s/he does not receive treatment, and not only what is likely to happen if s/he does receive treatment.* In other words, healthcare professionals should take into consideration the consequences of their omissions, as well as those of their actions. This might seem to go beyond professional obligations: clinicians might feel that they must assess the clinical benefits and risks *of therapies*, but that they are not responsible for what happens to people outside their clinics. Thus, for example, they may believe that they are responsible if they administer a drug, with the result that bone development or brain development is impaired. They may also believe that they are not equally responsible if the adolescent, against his/her professional advice, gets hormones in the streets or takes his or her life.

The extent to which all of us, including healthcare professionals, are responsible for the implications of our choices further down the line, or for what other people decide to do also as a result of our own choices, or of our own omissions, is open to debate. However, it is a mistake to believe that we bear no responsibility whatsoever for any of these implications. In this particular case, the problem is whether professionals are responsible for omitting to treat, as well as for treating, and for the consequences of their omissions. Omitting to treat, or deferring treatment, is not a morally neutral option. There are both ethical and legal grounds for considering carefully what would happen to the applicant *if s/he was not treated*, or treated later, or with hormones and in doses that s/he finds unhelpful.

6   ACTS AND OMISSIONS

Doctors are morally (and to some extent legally) responsible for the consequences of refusing to treat (see Chapter 7 for considerations relating to the law). They should therefore always consider what is likely to happen to people if they are refused treatment before deciding on whether to satisfy an applicant's request or not.

Doctors, generally speaking, do not have an obligation (either morally or legally) to treat just because a patient wants treatment, even if the applicant has the capacity to consent to treatment. Healthcare professionals (similarly to many other professionals) are entitled to refuse or withdraw their services. They can do so for moral reasons. Doctors are, for example, entitled, on the basis of conscientious objection, to refuse to perform abortions. However, in all cases the right not to treat is not absolute. For example, in the case of abortion, objecting doctors generally still need to intervene if the risks to the mother's health are serious and imminent.[35]

Healthcare professionals can also refuse to treat based on their clinical judgment. However, of course the doctor's and patient's opinions as to whether a certain treatment is harmful or beneficial may diverge, as it may happen in the case of administration of early treatment for gender dysphoria. These are precisely the instances in which the healthcare professional should also ponder the risks and benefits of treatment *versus non treatment*, because, both from a legal and an ethical point of view, failing to act is not necessarily a neutral or a safe option.

We shall discuss the law as it applies in England in Chapter 7, but it can be anticipated here that this is perhaps precisely the meaning of *Gillick*. The case of Gillick concerned the doctors' right to provide contraceptive advice and treatment to minors below the age of sixteen without involvement of parents (or of those with parental responsibility). Victoria Gillick, mother of three daughters, opposed to a circular distributed by the local authority to general practitioners authorising them to offer such services. Her arguments, based on her alleged right to know about their daughters' health and safety, failed the scrutiny of the courts. One of the main grounds for allowing doctors to provide contraceptive advice and treatment was that omissions, in many cases, could produce the worst consequences for the girls concerned. Lord Fraser argued that the doctor should meet the patient's request, provided that: "(1) that the girl. . . will understand his advice; (2) that he cannot persuade her to inform her parents. . .; *(3) that she is very likely to begin or continue having sexual intercourse with or without contraceptive treatment*; (4) that unless she receives contraceptive advice or treatment *her physical or mental health or both are likely to suffer*; (5) that her best interests require him to give her contraceptive advice or treatment or both without the parental consent".[36]

The final decision in Gillick was made also in view of the *consequences that were likely to occur if contraceptive advice and treatment were not given*: continuation of sexual intercourses without contraceptive, likely physical and/or mental suffering. This implies that there may be scope for the recognition of the doctors' responsibility for what can happen to patients or applicants *should they fail to administer requested treatment* (see Chapter 7). But perhaps more importantly, this reminds us all of the responsibilities that none of us can escape: when judging about what is good or right to do in any given circumstance, one should ponder the long term consequences of any choice that is open, including the choice of an omission.

The issue of whether we are *equally* responsible for our omissions as well as for our actions, and of *how responsible* we are for our omissions, is widely debated in ethics. If we are *equally* responsible for our omissions, this means that doctors who refuse to treat are responsible for what is likely to happen to the untreated child or adolescent in the same way that they are responsible for what is likely to happen if they provide treatment. It may be argued that doctors cannot share responsibility for what potential patients choose to do once they are refused treatment, sometimes against their advice. For example, doctors who judge the provision of hormones clinically unnecessary in any specific case cannot be held accountable if people obtain them from the illegal market, or cannot share criminal liability should turned down applicants get entangled in the justice system. This may seem to impose a too stringent responsibility on healthcare professionals.[37]

However, certainly inaction is not necessarily a 'morally safe place' to be. When we know that if we fail to do something, the consequences of our omissions are serious and potentially fatal for others, we have a stringent moral responsibility for those consequences. In fact, on Hall's account, the decision not to treat is best regarded as an action, not as an omission—and this would further explain in what sense doctors are responsible for not treating.[38]

In the case of gender dysphoria, practitioners may be reluctant to take responsibility for the act of starting treatment. Because the side effects of treatment are under scrutiny, doctors may feel that their *duty not to harm* (nonmaleficence) is best served by not taking the risks that may be associated with therapy. Given that they are dealing with children, they may feel a very strong responsibility not to subject them to any risk that they cannot foresee and therefore control, and may thus be inclined to postpone treatment until a later stage, in good faith that they are doing no harm and acting morally. Such a psychological reaction on the part of clinicians is understandable, but is not fully grounded, from an ethical point of view.

Omitting to treat at the right age may have a number of adverse and wide ranging consequences over the child's life, as has been shown before (see Chapter 5). Omitting treatment at prepubertal age means allowing a series of physical changes to occur when those changes are unwanted and are highly likely to have gravely adverse consequences when the adolescent continues to experience transsexualism. This is a harm that can be avoided by blocking pubertal changes and then administering cross sex hormones at the appropriate stage. Refusing to do so means bearing the moral responsibility for the consequences that the choice produces.

One final point should be noted on the issue of freedom not to treat. It could be argued that the claim that one has a right not to treat can only be sustained before a comparable freedom of patients to have quick access to alternative opinions and healthcare providers. It could be argued that if the patients do not have a right to quickly and flexibly access alternative healthcare providers, then doctors cannot ethically claim to have full freedom not to treat. It must be noted here that the National Healthcare System (NHS) that operates in the UK leaves scarce freedom of discretion to the users. The NHS decides who the treating clinician is. The decision of the therapist is alienated from the patient. This is especially problematic in delicate and intimate issues such as those relating to sex and gender. A successful outcome is largely dependent on mutual trust and respect, on mutual engagement in a therapeutic relationship. The possibility of a meaningful relationship can be seriously jeopardised by the fact that the individual has virtually no say and has to go to the clinic or to the specialist to whom s/he is referred. Should patients experience their treatment as dissatisfactory, or disagree with the clinician as to the therapeutic goals and methods of intervention, they have a very limited right to access alternative resources. They may get a second opinion, but again they *are referred* to a different specialist, and the choice is alienated from them. This highlights another crucial issue in the management of gender dysphoria: there are no alternative services in the UK to the Portman and Tavistock Clinic in London. This clinic is the only children's services clinic in the UK, and it established itself as the leading body of authority in the field, which implicitly regulates everyone else's clinical practice. Until 2011, the clinic has insisted on deferring treatment until at least Tanner Stage 4. Other endocrinologists in the country might have found it difficult to provide treatment to a patient who has been denied that treatment at the London clinic. In Chapter 7 we shall see that clinicians can and should treat minors in their best interests, but doctors outside what is the established specialist clinic in the country may find it somewhat intimidating to disagree with the clinical judgment of the practitioners operating in that clinic. In the UK, a doctor can be referred by other doctors to the General Medical Council (GMC—an independent regulator that has among its purposes that of securing proper standards of medical care) if there is a doubt that s/he failed to act according to established standards. An enquiry by the GMC may result in the suspension of the clinician from the Register of Medical Practitioners. If the doctor can prove that they acted according to sound, reasonable, and defensible clinical judgment (see Chapter 7 for more details), a claim is unlikely to succeed, but this would clearly be no fun process to go through.

Thus, of course, healthcare professionals should exercise their judgment, and this involves making individual judgments on individual patients' best interests. But the freedom of doctors to make these decisions can ethically be exercised if it is mutual, that is, if patients have got a corresponding freedom to choose as to whether that advice is sensible for them or not. Where patients have scant freedom to reasonably quickly access other services or providers, healthcare professionals have a more stringent responsibility to provide treatment.

So far, we have seen that there is no reason to believe that treatment of trans children and adolescents involves any undue interference with nature (or with God's will—an argument that should be left to the faith of each individual); there is no reason to assume that trans children cannot provide valid consent to treatment of their gender issues (especially in those cases in which the family supports them); finally, I have argued that early treatment is not unethical—indeed, it might be unethical not to provide it. There are further ethical and legal issues relating to the involvement of the family and determination of age of access to treatment. I will discuss the issues around family involvement in the next chapter, dedicated more precisely to the law. I shall now deal with determination of age of access to medical treatment.

7 AGEISM

The sixth version of the WPATH's *Standards of Care* stated clearly: "Any surgical intervention should not be carried out prior to adulthood, or prior to a real-life experience of at least two years in the gender role of the sex with which the adolescent identifies. The threshold of 18 should be seen as an eligibility criterion and not an indication in itself for active intervention".[39]

In the seventh version, the WPATH gives more specific guidelines relating to various types of surgery. For some surgery, such as a mastectomy, hormone therapy is not a requirement, and for some but not all surgery it is required that the patient has lived in a gender role congruent with gender identity for at least twelve continuous months (for example, for metoidioplasty or phalloplasty and vaginoplasty). For some but not all surgery the age of majority in a given country is also required.[40] The criteria of the sixth version have thus been somewhat tempered in the last version of the *Standards of Care*.

The Endocrine Society Guidelines have also corrected the previous strict age eligibility criterion. The relevant sections of these guidelines are reported in Box 6.1.

Box 6.1   Endocrine Society Guidelines: On Age of Access

5.1. We recommend that transsexual persons consider genital sex reassignment surgery only after both the physician responsible for endocrine transition therapy and the MHP find surgery advisable.

5.2. We recommend that genital sex reassignment surgery be recommended only after completion of at least 1 year of consistent and compliant hormone treatment.

5.3. We recommend that the physician responsible for endocrine treatment medically clear transsexual individuals for sex reassignment surgery and collaborate with the surgeon regarding hormone use during and after surgery.[41]

The dissent as to whether a fixed date for access to certain treatments is appropriate raises an important ethical issue about ageism. In principle, determination of a particular age of access to a certain treatment is ageist. There may be important clinical reasons to defer surgery for gender dysphoria after other stages of treatment, and only when in all likelihood the applicant is certain that irreversible changes should take place. When this point will be reached, however, cannot be determined *a priori*, and has to be a function of the development and of the maturity of the single individual.

Ageism is unjust discrimination by reason of age. Decisions regarding whether or not an applicant should receive treatment should not be based on age, but on the applicant's capacity to benefit from treatment. Capacity to benefit from treatment and capacity to provide valid consent are often a function of age, but this is not always the case. Indeed, in gender dysphoria capacity to benefit from treatment is often *inversely proportional to age*, in that it decreases as puberty advances.

The World Health Organization (WHO) and the United Nations (UN) have formally established that 'ageism', including ageism in healthcare provision, is unethical.[42] Discrimination based on age is a violation of one of the most fundamental human rights, the right to equality meant as nondiscrimination. According to the European Charter of Human Rights, age, together with sex, race, colour, ethnic or social origin, genetic features, language, religion or belief, political or any other opinion, membership of a national minority, property, birth, disability, and sexual orientation (Art. 21, Nondiscrimination) [43] is an arbitrary feature that does not justify difference in treatment.[44]

'Ageism' generally refers to the treatment of the older patient, and the declarations by the WHO and the UN are normally meant to protect the equal right of the older person to access medical treatment. However, younger people can be discriminated against based on age as well. Refusing to treat someone because s/he is too young is as unjust as refusing to treat someone because s/he is too old. Both are examples of discrimination based on age. Setting up age limits for access to treatment, in one direction or the other, is a form of ageism. Healthcare professionals need to provide valid reasons to refuse medical treatment: they need to show that the treatment is not in the best interests of the applicant. Appeal to age alone is ethically incongruent with ethical principles stated in virtually all conventions and declarations of human rights and fundamental freedoms.

Healthcare professionals could argue that it is irresponsible to treat children when the outcome of treatment is uncertain. However, if it is irresponsible and/or unethical to provide treatment whose risks and benefits are uncertain, then this is so *regardless of the age of the applicant*. Treating an adult would be as unethical as treating a child. The rationale for withholding treatment, if one has to be found, must be sought on other grounds and not on the basis of the age of the applicant.

In the closure of this chapter, it is opportune to mention another area of concern in the treatment of gender dysphoria, the Real Life Experience. This concerns adults more than children, in that Real Life Experience is clinically required before surgery takes place, which typically only occurs when the applicant is an adult. However, the Real Life Experience may take place during adolescence, or even in childhood for children treated with pubertal suppressant medications, and therefore it is worth considering in the context of the ethical issues associated with it.

8   ETHICAL AND CLINICAL ISSUES WITH THE REAL LIFE EXPERIENCE

It is accepted, and it is common clinical practice, to request trans who apply for irreversible treatment to undertake the so called Real Life Experience[45] (though it is to be noted that the latest version of the WPATH Standards of Care does not refer to Real Life Experience, but requests that "patients have lived continuously for at least 12 months in the gender role that is congruent with their gender identity" before genital surgery)[46]. As we have seen in Chapter 5, sometimes the Real Life Experience is also encouraged at earlier stages of treatment, when the child is administered pubertal suppressant medications. During this time, the applicant is advised to live socially as a person of the other gender, in order to explore whether they are more comfortable in that gender. The clinical reason for this is somehow obvious: with children, it is necessary to refine the diagnosis. With adults, before irreversible changes take place, the applicant needs to take any steps to avoid future dissatisfaction, and must verify as much as this is possible whether changing gender is highly likely to meet his or her expectations. Real Life Experience involves a spectrum of measures, ranging from cross dressing to adopting the body language, the mannerisms, and the roles one thinks or feels are appropriate for the desired gender.

Whereas the intention behind the Real Life Experience seems appropriate, it has been objected that insisting that applicants perform the Real Life Experience is likely to reinforce those very gender stereotypes that make surgery necessary for some. The Real Life Experience, thus, it has been argued, reinforces "social conformity by encouraging the individual to become an agreeable participant in a role-defined society, substituting one sex role stereotype for the other".[47]

There is certainly a valid point here. Gender minorities are not simply 'men trapped in women's bodies' and *vice versa*. The spectrum of genders and sexes is vast and must include various ways of expressing one's uniqueness. This stands for children as well as for adults. Channelling dissatisfaction into the blunt rejection of the gender roles associated with the assigned sex, and into the required adoption of the gender roles associated with the proposed or potential sex, may make little sense for two reasons: one is that gender minorities encompass a variety of ways of being. Treatment of gender minorities challenges the assumption that there are only two sexes and two genders, and that individuals who are not happy with one gender should necessarily be happy with the other. The other reason is that to the extent that the binary distinction of sex and gender is somehow responsible for the discomfort associated with atypical gender identification, the request of living in the life of the other gender risks reinforcing the binary distinction that is to a significant degree responsible for people's suffering.

There is another reason why the Real Life Experience raises ethical issues. People who are 'gender nomads', who do not conform to either one or the other gender, risk having to 'prove' their suitability for surgery by forcing themselves into roles that are not optimal for them, by therefore having to once more suffer pretending to be someone they are not and possibly 'deceiving' the healthcare professionals in order to obtain medical care. This endangers the therapeutic alliance that is needed for a successful outcome.

Importantly, the Real Life Experience risks exposing people who have not yet transitioned to social abuse. The Real Life Experience can be felt as a masquerade by both the individual and others in general, and given the strong social aversion to cross dressing, during the Real Life Experience gender minorities may be exposed to ridicule, verbal abuse, and further social stigma. It could be argued that such exposure is and must be a part of the Real Life Experience, if such an experience truly has to be real. In real life transsexuals *are* exposed to ridicule, abuse, and stigma, and those who choose to transition ought to be prepared to expose themselves to these. Whereas this can to some extent be correct, it is the role of medicine and society at large to prevent people from being exposed to such trauma; a balance must thus be found between allowing people to experience what it is to live in the other gender (including the experience of social ostracism, an experience that probably many trans already have) and preventing them from being harmed.

The problems inherent in the Real Life Experience are not necessarily reasons against the Real Life Experience altogether. Some kind of precaution in this sense before irreversible interventions take place is probably recommendable. However, as with all other parts of the care for gender minorities, the requirements cannot be unyielding, and must be tailored carefully to the individual's needs and to the social contexts in which they live.

The Real Life Experience must be an instrument for the patient to understand his or her gender(s), and for him or her to predict in what ways s/he will best adjust to the society in which s/he lives. It must not be imposed as a prerequisite for transition in some rigid format, and it must not primarily be a proof that the applicant is 'a true candidate' for surgery. The aim of the Real Life Experience must be to help the individual to explore his or her gender(s) and understand with the professionals what medical interventions can best serve his or her interests. This exploration cannot, of course, be imposed, but must encompass the patient's views and be based on a meaningful therapeutic alliance.

9 CONCLUSIONS

There are important ethical issues surrounding medical treatment for children with gender dysphoria. In this chapter I have analysed the major objections to such treatment, and I have shown that none of them provides a solid ground to deny access to early medical treatment.

The ethical decision making process encompasses four essential points:

1. Doctors have a *moral and legal* responsibility to consider broadly the children's welfare (see also Chapter 7).
2. Ethical analysis includes consideration not only of side effects of medications, but *likely consequences of treatment versus nontreatment*.
3. 'Consequences' include physical consequences, and also *psychological, social, and relational sequelae*.
4. Doctors are *morally responsible for decisions not to treat*.

On the basis of the clinical evidence discussed in Chapters 1–5, and of the ethical analysis performed so far, it can be concluded that there are no ethical grounds for deferring treatment until puberty is complete and the applicant is a young adult, because, at that stage, the damage caused by natural development might be difficult to undo. Indeed, it might be unethical not to treat as requested, if treatment is likely to prevent great harm and to save people's lives.

In the next chapter I will discuss some legal concerns relating to treatment of minors with gender issues.

KEY POINTS

- Treatment of trans minors raises a number of ethical dilemmas:

- *Playing God or fiddling with nature is unethical.*
- *We should change society, rather than mutilating children's bodies.*
- *It is unethical to experiment on children.*
- *Doctors should not expose children to potential harm.*

- None of these arguments stand rational scrutiny.
- Interfering with nature is a normal part of clinical practice.
- Society may need to change; yet gender dysphoric children may need to be treated medically.
- There is nothing unethical with experimental treatment *per se.*
- Doctors should not expose children to potential harm, and even less should they expose children to highly likely or real harm that can be prevented.
- Denying or deferring treatment to children with gender dysphoria may be unethical.

7 The Treatment of Minors with Gender Dysphoria
Legal Concerns

It is the judges who make the criminals [. . .] Punishment is a second-degree crime, which can show its face first. This is why societies are repressive: they are delegated to kill [. . .] They kill with Morality, itself sharp, but protected and guaranteed by procedure.

(*Jacques Brel*)[1]

Legalism is an abomination. I loathe it. You must remain anarchic.
(*Claude Cahun, Letter to André Breton c. 1953*)[2]

1 INTRODUCTION

Providing medical treatment should be in principle an easy procedure: even as children are concerned, in principle medical treatment should be given when it is good for the patient, or when it is bad for the patient not to receive it. Things are not so simple in practice. Healthcare professionals working with minors with Gender Identity Disorder (GID), and patients and families, may have concerns relating to their responsibilities and rights. In this chapter I address some of the legal concerns that may affect decisions about the treatment of minors with gender dysphoria. What is needed to secure consent for treatment so that the doctor does not face civil or even criminal liability? Can the minor, in particular, the transgender minor, have the capacity to consent to treatment? What is the role of the parents in securing consent? How should the best interests of the patient be assessed, and when might it be necessary to seek guidance from the courts? Could a refusal to treat be challenged in court, and in what circumstances should doctors be worried about liability in negligence both if they do and do not treat? The answers to these questions differ immensely from country to country. Even within the UK, England, Wales,[3] and Scotland have very different principles governing consent and minors or incapacitated adults. So it is not possible to set out any universal legal principles or address every country. There are even further legal hurdles relating to the position of children (and adults) with ambiguous sex and gender in society (for example, relating to registration at birth, documents such as passports, and so on). In England, the Gender Recognition Act 2004 has provided some answers relating to the rights and responsibilities of and towards transgender *adults*.[4] For reasons of space and consistency, I will only focus on some of the legal issues that are most likely to arise during the clinical encounter between healthcare professionals and minors with gender issues. I will in particular focus on Stage 1 treatment, which generally concerns people of less than sixteen years of age and which is perhaps the most controversial in many ways. What will be said, however, will clarify issues concerning older minors and even adults.

I seek first to use the Australian case of Alex to highlight some legal problems in this area. Then I examine in more detail each of the legal issues set out in the preceding and use English law to illustrate one set of answers. At a number of points I indicate how other jurisdictions may take a different approach to English law. I hope to argue that for the most part laws do not impede doctors in fulfilling their ethical duty to act in the best interests of the minor.

2 A CASE BEFORE THE COURTS

One of the first cases of transgender minors to appear before the courts is the one of *Alex*. The case concerned an Australian resident. The legal file narrates the long and heart breaking story of Alex,[5] who underwent a complex court case hearing, at the age of thirteen, to receive early medical treatment for GID. Alex had had a difficult upbringing, marked by parental rejection. Alex was registered as a female at birth and had a strong gender identification as a boy. Alex was looked after by an aunt. At school Alex refused to take part in activities with peers; he at times refused to drink for the whole duration of the school day in order to avoid going to the bathroom or wore a nappy. Alex was extremely distressed at the prospect of entering puberty. The aunt supported the transition to the other gender. The treatment Alex applied for was temporary suppression of pubertal development, in view of a later eventual administration of cross sex hormones. He was not seeking surgery at that stage. It was the first time that, in Australia, suspension of puberty was requested at such an early age. As doctors were concerned about the lawfulness of provision of treatment, the matter was brought before the courts. The courts authorised treatment.[6]

Let us now turn to the first issue outlined in the introduction: what is needed to secure consent for treatment.

3 HOW TO SECURE CONSENT

3.1 What Is *Consent?*

Consent is a process through which a patient agrees to a certain medical procedure. A doctor who, say, decided to provide treatment without consent would in normal circumstances be liable in the tort of trespass or in the crime of assault.[7] Consent is not simply an act of *assent*, but a process through which the patient (or those who are in the position to consent on his or her behalf—for example, those with parental responsibility, that is, normally the parents) acquires and understands the information material to the decision and agrees to what is being proposed.

Some extreme medical treatments may be contentious at law even in the presence of consent. One example is surgery for so called 'body dysmorphic disorder', where the patient feels an urge to have some healthy body parts amputated.[8] The case of surgery for GID has been considered in this light: it has been asked whether the unease with one's gender may be considered similar to the unease with healthy body parts that is seen in so called body dysmorphic disorder. In *Bellinger v. Bellinger* the House of Lords in England has accepted that the two conditions are of a different nature and has decided for the lawfulness of cross sex surgery.[9]

The modalities through which consent is gathered vary in different countries. In England, both in the NHS and in the private sector patients are normally required to sign a consent form.[10] Written consent forms are under English law one piece of evidence of what the patient has agreed to.[11]

3.2 When Is Consent Valid?

Consent is valid if three conditions are met: (1) the patient is acting *voluntarily*; (2) the patient is broadly aware of what s/he is consenting to (hence *informed* consent); (3) the patient has the *capacity to consent* to what is proposed.

With regard to condition 1, *voluntariness* refers to the patient acting without coercion and under no undue influence. It is generally rare for a patient "to be forced to acquiesce to medical treatment by a direct, coercive threat",[12] and in particular in our case it is unlikely that consent to the procedures sought by minors may be coerced by third parties. Much more relevant, instead, are conditions 2 and 3.

3.3 Information and Valid Consent

In order for consent to be valid the patient needs to be broadly aware of what s/he is consenting to. A doctor has a duty to give the patient careful advice and sufficient information enabling the patient to reach a rational decision. It is obvious that a doctor cannot spend an endless amount of time disclosing all information s/he has about the medical procedure at stake. It is likely that many patients would be unable to even understand and retain all that information. There is thus an issue of *how much information* and *what type of information* must be disclosed in order for consent to be valid. In England, it is established that a doctor should disclose the information in broad terms; normally the doctor should not disclose what a prudent patient would want to know,[13] but what a prudent doctor would hold appropriate to disclose.[14] With regard to the type of information, the doctor should provide in broad terms information about "the nature of the procedure which is intended",[15] the purposes of the procedure at stake, its main risks and benefits, and available alternatives. There should be evidence that the patient understands the information thus provided. Before a direct question by a patient, a doctor ought to answer truthfully even about the details that s/he would have otherwise omitted. No misrepresentation of the facts is lawful.[16] In our case, it is important that the doctor discloses the potential benefits but also the long term potential risks of treatment, including those that are not fully established (see Chapter 5). If the treatment is offered within a research study, further information needs to be provided to the patient, who is, in this case, also a research participant (see later in this chapter).

There are further issues. Can a minor give valid consent to suspension of puberty (or hormonal treatment) when s/he has not had the full experience of puberty itself (or of life in the other gender)? Does the patient need to have 'firsthand experience' in relation to the matter s/he is required to understand? In a case concerning an adult, the courts decided that such experience is not necessary for consent to be valid.[17]

Another question could be raised about the types of beliefs that could impinge upon the validity of consent.[18] Normally, if a patient makes a clinical decision based on a delusional belief, questions may be raised about the patient's understanding of the material facts. It could be asked whether the belief to be in the 'wrong body' may be considered delusional, akin to some psychotic beliefs.[19] Whereas there are cases reported in literature where the wish to change sex was a part of a delusional state,[20] it is accepted by the clinical community at large that transgenderism is not inherently linked to psychosis. The World Professional Association for Transgender Health (WPATH) *Standards of Care* read: "Phenomenologically, there is a qualitative difference between the presentation of gender dysphoria and the presentation of delusions or other psychotic symptoms. The vast majority of children and adolescents with gender dysphoria are not suffering from underlying severe psychiatric illness such as psychotic disorders".[21] In order to assess whether the patient has a delusion (that is, typically temporary even if recurrent) or a stable mismatch with the assigned gender, a careful clinical evaluation needs to be performed. Hence the importance, as we shall see later in this chapter, of a multidisciplinary clinical assessment. Finally, let us examine condition 3, capacity.

3.4   Capacity

One of the main concerns that healthcare professionals may have in treating children with gender dysphoria is whether these children have the legal capacity to request or to consent to medical treatment, particularly as treatment may commence at an early age (we have seen, Alex was thirteen years old, and in principle treatment could begin earlier—some children may reach Tanner Stage 2 at the age of nine). Even with young adolescents, capacity seems a concern of health professionals and professional bodies. For example, the WPATH *Standards of Care* read: "Feminizing/masculinizing hormone therapy may lead to irreversible physical changes. *Thus, hormone therapy should be provided only to those who are legally able to provide informed consent.* This includes people who have been declared by a court to be emancipated minors, incarcerated people, and cognitively impaired people who are considered competent to participate in their medical decisions".[22]

Capacity is interpreted differently in different countries, and likewise, capacity tests and the implications of declarations of incapacity may have different meanings.[23] I will consider here English law and I will focus specifically on how capacity applies to minors in the healthcare context.

Gillick v. West Norfolk and Wisbech Area Health Authority[24] provided an important characterisation of competence, or capacity, as it applies to minors. The *Gillick* case was a judicial review action initiated by the mother of five daughters of less than sixteen years of age. Victoria Gillick (the mother) argued that doctors could not lawfully provide contraceptive advice and treatment to girls under sixteen without the involvement of their parents. Mrs. Gillick's claim was unsuccessful. The House of Lords held by a majority "that the original advice circulated by the DHSS was not unlawful and that a child under sixteen can in certain circumstances give a valid consent to medical treatment, including contraception or abortion treatment, without parental knowledge or agreement".[25] *Gillick* established that a child under sixteen can give an effective consent to medical treatment providing that s/he had reached "sufficient understanding and intelligence to be capable of making up his own mind in the matter requiring decision".[26] This is known as the *Gillick* test, or *Gillick* competence test. It suggests that a mature child may have the capacity to consent to some examinations and treatment.[27] During the review there appeared to be disagreement on *what the child must be able to understand*. Lord Scarman argued that the child "must fully understand what is proposed including 'moral and family questions' and their emotional implications, whereas Lord Fraser only required the child to understand the doctor's advice".[28] Generally, the more serious the decision, the greater the capacity required of the minor; thus capacity may 'run out' when it comes to life threatening decisions.[29] In spite of disagreement, *Gillick* "establishes that a child below sixteen may lawfully be given general medical advice and treatment without parental agreement, provided that the child has achieved sufficient maturity to understand fully what is proposed. The doctor treating such a child on the basis of her consent alone will not be at risk of either a civil action or criminal prosecution".[30] Although the implications of *Gillick* in terms of children's right to autonomy are discussed,[31] '*Gillick* competence' is regarded as the landmark of adolescent autonomy in healthcare.[32]

Gillick was about provision of contraceptive advice and treatment; of course, this is hormonal treatment aimed at preventing greater harm and the long term adverse psychological and social consequences of nontreatment (see Chapter 5). In this respect, there are important similarities with hormonal treatment that can be provided to young transgenders. If hormonal treatment aimed at improving quality of life and preventing harm is ethically offered to minors in one case, there is no apparent reason why it should not be offered to minors in the other case as well. Suspension of puberty may involve more invasive hormonal treatment than contraception. However, untreated gender variance has arguably more severe and varied consequences over a child's welfare than lack of contraception, and whereas those who are refused hormonal contraception can easily opt for alternative contraceptive methods, there are no alternatives for transgender youth, except for the illegal market and unqualified medical help or medical tourism in the best scenario.

It should be noted that the issue of capacity has been widely discussed in the English courts. A definition of capacity is now provided by the Mental Capacity Act 2005 (MCA). This applies to people aged sixteen and above. Box 7.1 cites the relevant parts of sections 2 and 3 of the MCA.

Box 7.1   Mental Capacity Act 2005, Sections 2 and 3

2. People Who Lack Capacity

(1) For the purposes of this Act, a person lacks capacity in relation to a matter if at the material time he is unable to make a decision for himself in relation to the matter because of an impairment of, or a disturbance in the functioning of, the mind or brain.
(2) It does not matter whether the impairment or disturbance is permanent or temporary.
(3) A lack of capacity cannot be established merely by reference to—
    a. A person's age or appearance, or
    b. A condition of his, or an aspect of his behaviour, which might lead others to make unjustified assumptions about his capacity.

3. Inability to Make Decisions

(1) For the purposes of section 2, a person is unable to make a decision for himself if he is unable—
    a. To understand the information relevant to the decision
    b. To retain that information
    c. To use or weigh that information as part of the process of making the decision, or
    d. To communicate his decision (whether by talking, using sign language or any other means)
(2) A person is not to be regarded as unable to understand the information relevant to a decision if he is able to understand an explanation of it given to him in a way that is appropriate to his circumstances (using simple language, visual aids or any other means).
(3) The fact that a person is able to retain the information relevant to a decision for a short period only does not prevent him from being regarded as able to make the decision
(4) The information relevant to a decision includes information about the reasonably foreseeable consequences of—
    a. deciding one way or another, or
    b. failing to make the decision.[33]

3.4.1 *Capacity and Refusal of Treatment*

The application for treatment for gender dysphoria raises an issue of *consent* to treatment and not one of *refusal of treatment*. However, it is worth mentioning that whereas minors may under English law have a right *to consent* to medical treatment, they may at the same time *not* have the right to refuse it. The recognition of a child's right to consent to a certain medical treatment does not automatically imply the recognition of that child's right to refuse the same medical treatment. When an adult has the required legal capacity,[34] s/he acquires an absolute right to refuse medical treatment, independently of the outcome and apparent rationality of the decision.[35] Similar provisions are in force in many liberal states. For example, Art. 32 of the Italian Constitution reads: "Nobody can be forced into medical treatment, unless it is so disposed by law". If a doctor violates this constitutional rule, s/he may be liable for assault, fraudulent damage, or manslaughter, according to the circumstances, under Art. 610 of the Penal Code.

For minors things are not as stark. The equilibrium between capacity to consent and capacity to refuse treatment is a delicate one, which depends on the combination of case law and statutes (the Children Act 1989, for example, allows mature minors to refuse medical or psychiatric treatments in defined circumstances).[36] Very broadly, it can be affirmed that under English law the competent minor does not necessarily have the same absolute right to refuse medical treatment as the competent adult. A discussion of the laws on refusal of treatment in minors goes beyond the remit of this book,[37] as we are primarily concerned here with access to medical treatment.

4 CAN CHILDREN WITH GENDER DYSPHORIA HAVE THE CAPACITY TO CONSENT TO TREATMENT FOR THEIR GENDER ISSUES? THE PROBLEM OF MENTAL ILLNESS

GID is currently classified as a mental illness (see Chapter 4). Mental illness can be believed to jeopardise the sufferer's decision making capacity, in particular, capacity to make decisions about treatment for the illness itself (this reasoning could, of course, be also applied to an adult). The assumption that mental illness subverts people's capacity is one that recurs in ordinary discourses as well as in part of the scientific literature.[38] As it will be suggested in Chapter 8, there are grounds for challenging the classification of transgenderism as a mental illness. But even if transgenderism was appropriately regarded as a mental illness, this would not *ipso facto* entail patient incapacity to make decisions about medical treatment. Since the 1990s in England it has been accepted that the presence of a mental disorder does not necessarily affect capacity to make decisions about medical and psychiatric treatment, including treatment for the mental illness.[39] In the specific case of treatment for gender dysphoria, it cannot be assumed that a patient (whether minor or adult) with gender dysphoria lacks capacity to consent to treatment *because of his or her condition*. It should be acknowledged that the experience of the child and what the child has to say are essential both to understanding the degree of his or her predicaments and to framing useful strategies of intervention.[40] It is noted that trans children often suffer anxiety and depression, which may be thought to jeopardise their decision making capacity, which could push them to request perhaps unnecessary treatment. However, anxiety and depression are usually secondary to gender dysphoria, and "often arise during puberty as a consequence of the distress that accompanies their bodily changes. For many adolescents, being refused treatment during this difficult period is a form of psychological torture".[41] Therefore, whereas the child may need assistance in assessing the therapeutic options open to him or her, it cannot be assumed that s/he lacks capacity because s/he suffers from what is currently (and, I will argue, misleadingly) classified as a mental illness.

5   CAN CHILDREN WITH GENDER DYSPHORIA HAVE THE CAPACITY TO CONSENT TO TREATMENT FOR THEIR GENDER ISSUES? THE PROBLEM OF YOUNG AGE

The first stage of therapy, in order to be effective, should begin early in puberty, and it can be asked whether young minors sometimes of the age of twelve or thirteen can have the required capacity to make decisions on treatment that has significant effects on their development. It can be asked how a child can have the capacity to consent to suppression of puberty, if puberty is something that they have not yet experienced. It can also be asked how a child can have sufficient insight to decide that the gender of rearing is mistaken, if s/he has not yet experienced what it is to be that gender. There are two separate issues here: one is whether younger minors can have the capacity to consent to treatment; the other is whether children who have not yet experienced puberty can be capable of deciding to have that puberty suppressed.

On the first point, capacity "does not depend on the age of the child, but on subjective features of the child in respect to the particular treatment proposed".[42] The British Medical Association (BMA) highlights that "both law and ethics stress that the views of children and young people must be heard",[43] and "this is the message of the Children Act 1989 and its equivalents in Scotland and Northern Ireland".[44]

The BMA has offered useful guidelines in this respect. These guidelines are not the law, but they summarise key points of good clinical practice, in respect of the law. These are reported in Box 7.2.

Box 7.2   BMA Guidelines: Children Should

- Be kept as fully informed as possible about their care and treatment
- Be able to expect health professionals to act as their advocates
- Have their views and wishes sought and taken into account as part of promoting their welfare in the widest sense
- Be presumed able to make their own treatment decisions when they have sufficient 'understanding and intelligence'
- Be encouraged to take decisions in collaboration with other family members, especially parents, if this is feasible.[45]

The BMA insists on establishing a good communication as a fundamental part of a relationship of trust and respect between child and professional, which is essential to a good outcome. Children should not be excluded from decision making, and including them should be the norm. Children should not be regarded as incompetent just because they do not agree with the physicians. Importantly, doctors should not judge the capacity of a child solely on the basis of his or her age.

In other international documents, similar points are made. For example, the Convention on the Rights of the Child, adopted in 1989 by the UN General Assembly, states that the child has a right to have his or her views accorded due weight in relation to the child's maturity (Article 12).[46] Thus, whereas children are not automatically presumed to have capacity, it is an important principle of ethics, law, and good clinical practice that they are not automatically assumed to lack capacity, and that therefore a therapeutic relationship be based on taking seriously into consideration the child's opinions about his or her own care.

Let us turn on the second point: doctors may question whether a child who has not yet entered puberty can have the capacity to make the decision to have that puberty suppressed. Earlier in this chapter we have seen that, in England, the patient is not usually by law required to have 'firsthand experience' on the matter of deliberation in order for consent to be valid. A child who enters puberty may have sufficient knowledge of him- or herself to know that puberty in the gender of assignment does not match his or her gender identity. Gender, in fact, is not acquired at puberty; gender expectations accompany the child since birth or even before (see Chapter 3). It could be objected that only after having experienced puberty can a person know that they are transgender. For this reason, clinical guidelines insist that the child has *some* experience of puberty in his or her 'biological sex' before medical treatment begins, and the reaction of the child to the 'spontaneous' pubertal changes is still used diagnostically (see Chapter 5). This, however, does not mean that a child must have a *full experience* of puberty before treatment may begin. We have seen earlier in the book that by the age of six or seven sex typing is complete, and atypical gender identification may be evident in young children. By the age of entering puberty, often a diagnosis may already be reasonably made, and early treatment can also assist in making an accurate diagnosis. A fine balance between using 'spontaneous development' and suspension of puberty to understand and cope with the child's predicaments must thus be found in the therapeutic relationship with each individual child.

Let us now see how consent should be gathered. I will make some general observations first, and then examine the specific case of early treatment for gender dysphoria.

6   CONSENT TO TREATMENT: THE ROLE OF THE FAMILY

The Family Law Reform Act 1969, in force in England and Wales, at section 8 states that a minor who has attained the age of sixteen can give valid consent to any surgical, medical, or dental treatment. "Surgical, medical or dental treatment includes any procedure undertaken for the purposes of diagnosis, and this section also applies to any procedure (including the administration of an anaesthetic) that is ancillary to that treatment".[47] Where a minor has by virtue of section 8 given effective consent, it shall not be necessary to obtain consent from the parents or guardian. However, there is an obligation on doctors to attempt to persuade the minor to inform the parents or allow him or her to do so.[48] This seems to imply that a sixteen- or seventeen-year-old minor who applies for treatment for gender dysphoria should in principle be able to proceed with therapy, give valid consent to it, and have a right to confidentiality, if the treatment appears in his or her best interests, even if this goes against the judgment of the parents or of those with parental responsibility. Younger children could also in principle provide consent to medical treatment on their own, if they are *Gillick competent*.[49]

International guidelines, instead, insist on the importance of the family/guardian's consent. We have discussed this in Chapter 5, but it is worth repeating it here in this context. WPATH, as we saw previously, states: "Adolescents may be eligible for puberty suppressing hormones as soon as pubertal changes have begun. In order for the adolescents *and their parents to make an informed decision* about pubertal delay, it is recommended that the adolescents experience the onset of puberty to at least Tanner Stage Two" [50] (my emphasis). WPATH also recommends: "Adolescents may be eligible to begin feminizing/masculinizing hormone therapy, *preferably with parental consent*. In many countries, 16-year-olds are legal adults for medical decision-making and do not require parental consent. Ideally, treatment decisions should be made among the adolescent, the family, and the treatment team".[51]

There may be cogent reasons why the international guidelines stress the importance of parental participation. Treatment for gender dysphoria is complex and involves others so much that it would be effectively difficult to treat a child against the parents' or carers' wishes and to maintain confidentiality. Experts agree that "adolescents need the support of their parents in this complex phase of their lives".[52] "Mental health professionals can play an important role by educating people in these settings regarding gender nonconformity [. . .]. This role may involve consultation with school counsellors, teachers, and administrators, human resources staff, personnel managers and employers, and representatives from other organizations and institutions".[53] Certainly gender transition involves a wide circle (for example, the school), and it is unlikely that a child alone would be able to cope with all the modifications in his or her life without the support of carers.

Despite this, it is probably misleading to assume that doctors have a legal obligation to abide to the letter to the clinical guidelines. WPATH itself recognises that clinical guidelines can be modified "because of a patient's unique anatomic, social, or psychological situation [. . .] or the need for specific harm reduction strategies".[54] In the context of gathering valid consent, a veto *a priori* against treatment without parental consent is difficult to justify. Unless it can be shown that parental consent is *always* essential to the child's welfare, healthcare professionals should be open to the possibility—albeit remote—of treating minors with gender dysphoria without parental consent. It cannot be assumed that parents always serve or even understand their children's best interests, and the decision to treat should ultimately be made in the best interests of the child. As Lord Scarman argued in *Gillick*, "parental rights exist only so long as they are needed for the protection of the person and property of the child".[55] In the unfortunate and possibly rare cases in which parental support is unavailable, clinicians should assess whether *not receiving treatment* is ultimately better for the competent applicant than being treated without parental support.[56] There is a further reason why it may be prudent to obtain parental consent for early medical treatment for gender dysphoria.

7 CONSENT TO PARTICIPATION IN RESEARCH: THE ENGLISH APPROACH

The Tavistock and Portman Clinic in London, the UK clinic providing treatment for children with gender dysphoria, on 6 April 2011 published the news that it will begin a research study of the effects of 'blockers' early in puberty, declaring that the study has received the approval of the National Research Ethics Services.[57] Thinking of early treatment for gender dysphoria as *medical research* has a number of consequences.

A first consequence is the impact on the process of gathering consent. The Royal College of Paediatrics and Child Health states that a *Gillick* competent child can consent to participation in research.[58] However, things may be more complicated than this. *Gillick* was not about participation in research, and section 8 of the Family Law Reform Act 1969 deals with therapeutic and diagnostic procedures, not with participation in research. It is thus not clear that *Gillick* or the Family Law Reform Act 1969 would apply to research. Pattinson warns that "doctors relying on this guidance [on the guidance offered by the Royal College of Paediatrics and Child Health] would be well advised to take special caution before reaching the conclusion that a child whose consent they wish to rely on has the requisite maturity and understanding".[59] Mason and Laurie argue that it is generally more prudent of doctors to obtain the consent of the parents before experimental treatment is provided, even if the minors were found to have the legal capacity to provide consent.[60].

Another consequence of thinking of a medical intervention as medical research relates to the modalities in which the therapy is administered within a research study. Specific provisions regulate the modalities in which research involving children should take place. An examination of the laws regulating participation of minors to clinical research goes beyond the remit of this book, but a few considerations are necessary. Two European Directives, the Clinical Trials Directive 2001 and Good Clinical Practice (GCP) Directive 2005,[61] have significantly shaped the law on clinical research.[62] The Clinical Trials Directive 2001 has been transposed into law in the UK by the Medicine for Human Use (Clinical Trials) Regulations 2004. "The aim of the Directive is to simplify and harmonise the regulation of clinical trials. There are two main aspects to this: the establishment of a clear procedure for dealing with clinical trials and the facilitation of effective co-ordination of clinical trials throughout Europe".[63] In the UK, the government has also decided that, in 2011, a new health research regulatory agency should be created. "This new regulator is to have at its core the overarching body for the NHS Research Ethics Committees in England: the National Research Ethics Services".[64] Schedule 1 of the regulations deals with consent to participation in research. "As far as children are concerned, the Schedule provides for a hierarchy of consent on behalf of the child, commencing with a parent or person with parental responsibility. The others are personal legal representatives and professional legal representatives (i.e. someone nominated by the relevant health care provider) but consent can only be taken from these in emergencies".[65] If the research study is regulated by the Clinical Trials Regulations 2004, then the consent of someone with parental responsibility will be *necessary*.[66]

What happens if the parents are unwilling to consent to treatment for their child? If the research study is not regulated by the Clinical Trials Regulations 2004, whether or not doctors can lawfully proceed based on the minor's consent alone, Mason and Laurie seem to suggest, depends on whether the procedure is therapeutic or not, and on the severity of the procedure.[67] If the research study is regulated by the Clinical Trials Regulations 2004, the regulations provide for a professional legal representative. The regulations provide that the participant's doctor can also consent on behalf of the child, if s/he is not connected with the conduct of the trial.[68] Schedule 1 of the Clinical Trials Regulations 2004 contains the Conditions and Principles which apply to all Clinical Trials (Part 2) and Conditions and Principles which apply in Relation to a Minor (Part 4). See Boxes 7.3 and 7.4.[69]

Box 7.3   Clinical Trials Regulation, Schedule 1, Part 4: Conditions and Principles which Apply to All Clinical Trials

1. Clinical Trials shall be conducted in accordance with the ethical principles that have their origin in the Declaration of Helsinki, and that are consistent with good clinical practice and the requirements of these regulations.
2. Before the trial is initiated, foreseeable risks and inconveniences have been weighed against the anticipated benefit for the individual trial subject and other present and future patients.
3. The rights, safety, and well-being of the trial subjects are the most important considerations and shall prevail over interests of science and society.
4. The available non-clinical and clinical information on an investigational medicinal product shall be adequate to support the clinical trial.
5. Clinical trials shall be scientifically sound, and described in a clear, detailed protocol.
6. A trial shall be conducted in compliance with the protocol that has a favourable opinion from an ethics committee.
7. The medical care given to, and medical decisions made on behalf of, subjects shall always be the responsibility of an appropriately qualified doctor or, when appropriate, of a qualified dentist.
8. Each individual involved in conducting a trial shall be qualified by education, training, and experience to perform his or her respective task(s).
9. Subject to the other provisions of this schedule relating to consent, freely given informed consent shall be obtained from every subject prior to clinical trial participation.
10. All clinical trial information shall be recorded, handled, and stored in a way that allows its accurate reporting, interpretation, and verification.
11. The confidentiality of records that could identify subjects shall be protected respecting the privacy and confidentiality rules in accordance with the requirements of the Data Protection Act 1998 and the law relating to confidentiality.
12. Investigational medicinal product used in the trial shall be (a) manufactured or imported, and handled and stored, in accordance with the principles and guidelines of good manufacturing practice, and (b) used in accordance with the approved protocol.
13. Systems with procedures that assure the quality of every aspect of the trial shall be implemented.

Conditions Based on Article 3 of the Directive

14. A trial shall be initiated only if an ethics committee and the licensing authority comes to the conclusion that the anticipated therapeutic and public health benefits justify the risks and may be continued only if compliance with this requirement is permanently monitored.
15. The rights of each subject to the physical and mental integrity, to privacy, and to the protection of the data concerning him in accordance with the Data Protection Act 1998 are safeguarded.
16. Provision has been made for insurance or indemnity to cover the liability of the investigator and sponsor which may arise in relation to the clinical trial.

Box 7.4   Clinical Trials Regulation, Schedule 1, Part 4: Conditions and
Principles which Apply in Relation to a Minor

Conditions

1. A person with parental responsibility for the minor or, if by reason of the emergency nature of the treatment provided as part of the trial no such person can be contacted prior to the proposed inclusion of the subject in the trial, a legal representative for the minor has had an interview with the investigator, or another member of the investigating team, in which he has been given the opportunity to understand the objectives, risks, and inconveniences of the trial and the conditions under which it is to be conducted.
2. That person or legal representative has been provided with a contact point where he may obtain further information about the trial.
3. That person or legal representative has been informed of the right to withdraw the minor from the trial at any time.
4. That person or legal representative has given his informed consent to the minor taking part in the trial.
5. That person with parental responsibility or the legal representative may, without the minor being subject to any resulting detriment, withdraw the minor from the trial at any time by revoking his informed consent.
6. The minor has received information according to his capacity of understanding, from staff with experience with minors, regarding the trial, its risks, and its benefits.
7. The explicit wish of a minor who is capable of forming an opinion and assenting the information referred to in the previous paragraph to refuse participation in, or to be withdrawn from, the clinical trial at any time is considered by the investigator.
8. No incentives or financial inducements are given—(a) to the minor; or (b) to a person with parental responsibility for that minor or, as the case may be, the minor's legal representative, except provision for compensation in the event of injury or loss.
9. The clinical trial relates directly to a clinical condition from which the minor suffers or is of such a nature that it can only be carried out on minors.
10. Some direct benefit for the group of patients involved in the clinical trial is to be obtained from that trial.
11. The clinical trial is necessary to validate data obtained—(a) in other clinical trials involving persons able to give informed consent, or (b) by other research methods.
12. The corresponding scientific guidelines of the European Medicine Agency are followed.

(continued)

Box 7.4   (continued)

Principles

13. Informed consent given by a person with parental responsibility or a legal representative to a minor taking part in a clinical trial shall represent the minor's presumed will.
14. The clinical trial has been designed to minimise pain, discomfort, fear, and any other foreseeable risk in relation to the disease and the minor's stage of development.
15. The risk threshold and the degree of distress have to be specially defined and constantly monitored.
16. The interests of the patient always prevail over those of science and society.

8   IS THERE A RIGHT TO OBTAIN *INVESTIGATIONAL* THERAPIES?

In England, the case of *Burke* established that people generally have no right to obtain medical treatment that is judged by the doctor to be against their best interest.[70] We shall discuss this at a greater length shortly. The cases of *Simms v. Simms*, *R (Rogers) v. Swindon PCT* and *R (Gordon) v. Bromley PCT* raised the issue of whether patients may have a right to obtain experimental treatments.[71] *Simms v. Simms* concerned the use of invasive brain surgery for variant Creutzfeldt-Jakob disease, a neuro-degenerative disease sometimes called 'mad cow disease' that invariably leads to progressive illness and premature death.[72] The treatment at stake had been used routinely for other conditions, such as thrombosis, but had not been tested for this disease. There was no other possible treatment for this condition. The patients in this case were eighteen and sixteen years old. The parents requested the treatment on their children's behalf, and there was a consultant neurosurgeon willing to provide it. In authoris-ing the treatment P. Butler-Sloss took into consideration the unquantifi-able benefit, but also the lack of alternative treatments. Obtaining the treatment in question, even if to some extent experimental, may be in the best interests of the patients (including the minor patients) "where participation [in the research study] is the only way of getting a chance to receive innovative treatment for an otherwise untreatable condition".[73] The courts thus *authorised* treatment: it is important to note that they did not *oblige* an unwilling doctor to provide it. This case is important because it reiterates the principle, accepted generally, that experimental treatment (or what is classified as such) can on occasions be the best bet, even when given to minors or incapacitated adults. This case also stresses that it is at times important to evaluate not only potential risks of *the treatment at stake*, but also the potential risks of *not* providing it. Somehow, this reconnects us with the discussion on acts and omissions, made in Chapter 6. The courts' decision in *Simms* reminds us that when assessing the clinical options open, it is necessary to look at what would happen to people if the treatment they request were not provided, and, therefore, at the foreseeable consequences of *omissions* of treatment, not just at the foreseeable consequences of provision of treatment.

The cases of *Rogers* and *Gordon* went somewhat differently. These cases also concerned the provision of experimental treatment, but the Primary Care Trust (PCT) was *unwilling* to provide it; in both cases the patients sought judicial review on the grounds that the decision was arbitrary; irrational; and, in *Rogers*'s case, failed to give proper consideration to the relevant facts. In both cases, the review was in the patients' favour, and their request was referred back to the PCT for reconsideration. As we shall see later in this chapter, if a patient with gender dysphoria were to be denied medical treatment, one option would be to apply for judicial review. There is one further issue to examine, namely, whether it is appropriate to consider Stage 1 treatment for gender dysphoria as *experimental* or whether it should be administered only within a research study.

9   INNOVATIVE TREATMENT OR RESEARCH?

As explained in Chapter 5, there are aspects relating to the GnRHa that are under investigation. A question thus arises as to whether this treatment should be provided only within a research study. Stauch, Wheat, and Tingle define *research* as "any systematic inquiry aimed at discovering new facts about the way things in the world around us behave. In the case of medical research, the object of such inquiry is usually improving the efficacy of medical treatments. This includes the development of new forms of treatment and the ways in which medical treatments can be more effectively administered".[74] From this wide perspective, early treatment for gender dysphoria can be classed as *medical research*. However, a distinction is usually made between *innovative treatment* and *medical research*. The distinction sometimes refers to the case of *Simms v. Simms* discussed in the preceding.[75] It is worth repeating here the quotation cited already: "where participation [in the research study] is the only way of getting a chance to receive *innovative treatment* for an otherwise untreatable condition".[76] A question arises as to whether early treatment for gender dysphoria is best classed as (therapeutic) medical research or *innovative treatment*.

The distinction between the two usually lies with the *intention* of the healthcare professional. The primary aim of *medical research* "is to produce new knowledge for the benefit of future patients; the primary aim of medical treatment is to benefit the immediate patient".[77] Insofar as the primary aim of early treatment for gender dysphoria is to benefit the immediate patient, there is a ground to perhaps enclose it under the umbrella of *innovative treatments*. Yet, insofar as the medical intervention produces "generalisable knowledge related to human health or medical treatment",[78] it is perhaps also plausible to consider it as *medical research*. Therefore, early treatment for gender dysphoria could be placed at the interface between innovative treatment and research.

This distinction, it has been argued, is particularly important in order to protect patients from so called "therapeutic misconception",[79] where participants may believe that the treatment may benefit them, when the primary purpose of their participation is to gather information that will not be directly beneficial to them. The distinction is also important because categorising an intervention as treatment, although innovative, could "be used to justify a lower level of legal protection on levels of information and disclosure of risks than those appropriate for research, notwithstanding the fact that the effects and risks of an innovative or experimental procedure by definition are yet to be proven".[80] The distinction, thus, is therefore apparently meant to offer special protection to the patients.

However, it is worth noting that none of the most well established guidelines on the treatment for gender dysphoria suggests that early stages of treatment are to be regarded as experimental or are to be provided within a research study (see the guidelines discussed Chapter 5). They set the standards for *clinical practice*, not for clinical research. The difference may be subtle, but it is nonetheless important. Providing treatment only within a research study, in fact, not only may restrict access to the therapies (for example, to patients able to be monitored in the longer term or to patients whose parents are willing to consent to therapy); it may also restrict accessibility to alternative healthcare providers. I will return to this later. Before this, we need to discuss the notion of best interests: in principle, a team of specialists should be able to provide treatment in the interests of a minor, following the guidelines established by competent authorities, which will be further discussed in the following.

10 BEST INTERESTS: WHAT ARE THEY?

Section 1 of the Children Act 1989 states that the welfare of the child must be the "paramount consideration".[81] The BMA also states: "The welfare of children and young people is the paramount consideration in decisions about their care".[82] How are the child's best interests determined, and who decides? These two questions are very much intertwined. Who decides on the child's best interests depends on how these interests are understood. Traditionally, in English jurisprudence best interests have been considered narrowly as *medical* interests. Thus generally, best interests (those of adults as well) have been decided on the basis of the *medical* opinion: this is known as the *Bolam* test.[83] Essentially, *Bolam* established that a doctor's conduct is acceptable if it conforms to a responsible body of medical opinion, even if a different body of medical opinion holds a different or contrary view. In stating this, effectively the courts delegated to the medical profession the determination of best interests; neither the judges nor even the patients themselves would in principle be arbiters of their best interests, under the spirit of *Bolam*. It would be up to the doctor to decide, and his or her decision would have been difficult to challenge, insofar as an expert witness could be found who would have chosen the same line of action as the doctor in question.

The significance of *Bolam* has been tempered by a later case, *Bolitho*. In this case the courts established that the professional opinion also needs to be *reasonable or responsible*, and not just conform to 'the skilled and competent professional' standard. This in practice means that it is not enough to do what some other, or many others, would do in the given circumstances. It was stated:

> The court has to be satisfied that the exponents of the body of opinion relied on can demonstrate that such opinion has a logical basis. In particular, in cases involving as they so often do, the weighing up of risks against benefits, the judge before accepting a body of opinion as being reasonable, responsible or respectable, will need to be satisfied that, in forming their views, the experts have directed their minds to the questions of comparative risks and benefits and have reached a defensible conclusion on the matter.[84]

The judge in *Bolitho* stated: "if in a rare case, it can be demonstrated that the professional opinion is not capable of withstanding logical analysis, the judge is entitled to hold that the body of opinion is not reasonable or responsible".[85] Later cases, such as *A v. A Health Authority* also established other important elements relating to the determination of best interests:[86] best interests cannot be intended narrowly as medical interests, but must encompass a "range of ethical, social, moral, emotional and welfare considerations".[87] In *A Hospital NHS Trust v. S and others* it was stated:[88] "When considering the best interests of a patient, it is [. . .] the duty of the court to assess the advantages and disadvantages of the various treatment and management options, the viability of each such option and the likely effect each would have on the patient's best interests and, I would add, his enjoyment of life [. . .] any likely benefit of treatment has to be balanced and considered in the light of any additional suffering the treatment option would entail".[89]

When it is not immediately evident what is in a patient's best interests, or when there is a dispute between the interested parties (for example, the family and the healthcare professionals), it will be up to the courts to determine the patient's best interests and no longer up to the doctors alone. The courts will be now guided by the MCA 2005, in particular Part I, for what concerns people aged sixteen and above where there is a question as to the patient's capacity to determine his or her own best interests.[90] The act does not define *best interests*, but insists on the fact that they encompass not only medical interests, but also the person's present and past feelings, wishes, beliefs, and values. In all cases, and thus in cases of younger minors as well, best interests will be assessed in light not only of medical evidence, but also of the non-medical evidence relating to the patient's overall condition.[91] In the UK, the General Medical Council (which, it should be mentioned here, is not the law in the UK) also states that the child's best interests are not confined to clinical interests but include, among other factors, the views and values of the child, of the parents, and an evaluation of the choice, if there is more than one, which will least restrict the child's future options.[92]

10.1   Determination of Best Interests in Trans Minors: How the Doctors Should Proceed

Of course, determination of the child's best interests may not be straightforward. The main problem with best interests is that they are not always objective—what is in my best interests might not be in yours. Therefore, what counts as someone's best interests is debatable and sometimes negotiable. In the case of transgender minors, determination of best interests is perhaps even more complicated in that it encompasses *the prediction of the outcome of gender dysphoria*. This prediction cannot be made solely based on the expressed feelings of the applicants. This, as we saw in Chapter 5, is something that the clinical community is acutely aware of. The differentiation of desisters and persisters is a crucial issue, given that persisters will benefit from medical treatment and desisters may not: they may be false positives. However, it should be noted that even desisters may benefit from early treatment. As we saw in Chapter 5, early suspension of puberty may allow the child the time to explore his or her gender without the fear of growing in the 'wrong' body, and may actually *prevent* the later provision of more irreversible treatments (such as hormones) to false positives. If treatment is withheld, instead, or postponed, the child who is a persister will incur certain and preventable harm. This means that whereas in other situations it may be prudent to defer medical treatment until the child is older and more mature, delaying treatment of even a few months in cases of gender dysphoria may have hideous consequences.

Where does this leave healthcare professionals? Of course, healthcare professionals cannot be expected to be clairvoyants. All that can be expected of them is to make a careful assessment of each individual applicant, by involving, wherever possible and appropriate, the family, in order to understand the history and the extent of the child's discomfort and to make a prediction that is as accurate as possible. In the clinics that adopt a combined approach, as we have seen in Chapter 5, generally the child is seen by a team of specialists, as gender dysphoria encompasses endocrinological, psychological, and social issues. (It should be noted that WPATH in 2011 has taken a flexible approach and contemplates the possibility that individual healthcare professionals be involved with patients with gender dysphoria. WPATH also allows for individual health professionals to modify the clinical guidelines to suit the needs of the individual patient. These departures, WPATH warns, should be recognised as such, explained to the patient, and documented through informed consent.[93]) If the specialists, after careful evaluation, regard the dysphoria as strong and likely to persist, and if deferring treatment seems on balance of probabilities the most risky option, then there is a ground for considering early treatment as being in the best interests of the child. Determination of best interests should also be based on best available clinical evidence and on published research (evidence-based medicine). If healthcare professionals assess the child's best interests in this manner and it appears that initiating treatment seems, on balance, in the best interests of the particular child, they should be able to commence treatment and their conduct will be most likely irreprehensible.[94]

11   COULD A DOCTOR BE HELD NEGLIGENT FOR TREATING OR FOR NOT TREATING A CHILD WITH GENDER DYSPHORIA?

Doctors may worry that if they offer early treatment to minors they could expose themselves to allegations of malpractice. What if a patient at a later stage complained? Conversely, would they be liable in negligence if they fail to treat? Could patients who have been refused treatment claim that the doctor has been negligent? It would be very difficult for an applicant for gender treatment to succeed in a claim in negligence, at least in England, but let us see why this may be so.

In principle, healthcare professionals (as well as other categories of professionals) could be held negligent if:

1. They have a duty of care in a specific situation.
2. They have failed to meet the standard of care that is expected and up to current standards.
3. There is a causal connection between the damage or harm to the plaintiff (the patient making the claim) and the defendant's (the doctor's) careless conduct.
4. The damage is not unforeseeable or too remote.

11.1   Duty of Care

Doctors must owe a duty of care to the patient in order to be liable in negligence. Sometimes the existence of a duty of care can be contested.[95] If a doctor agrees to treat a patient, then of course that doctor has a duty of care towards the patient. However, if a doctor sees a patient and then refuses to treat, as treatment, for example, is against his or her clinical judgment, the doctor has, in principle, no duty of care towards the patient and normally the courts will not intervene.[96] Therefore, if, for example, a trans child and the parents are seen by a specialist who, after evaluation, holds it premature or inappropriate for the child to receive treatment, the parents and the child typically have no grounds to claim that the doctor has breached his or her duty of care towards the child.[97] Put otherwise, in England, there is no duty to rescue.

In countries where a duty to rescue is established by law, such as in Italy or France, a doctor could in principle be held negligent for failing to see a patient or if, after seeing a patient, s/he fails to give a treatment, provided that harm or injury follows such refusal. In Italy, for example, articles 328, 591, and 593 of the Penal Code, respectively *Omission or Refusal of Official Acts*, *Abandonment of the Incapacitated*, and *Omission of Rescue*, establish a general duty to rescue falling on laypeople as well as on professionals. However, in principle, in countries where there is no established duty to rescue, negligence generally can only occur once the doctor has accepted the applicant as his or her own patient. It is only then that the doctor owes a duty of care to who has then become his or her patient.

However, according to Stauch, Wheat, and Tingle, there is an issue as to whether this may be questioned. They write:

> This question must now be considered in the light of the courts' obligation, under the Human Rights Act 1998, to develop common law in line with rights under the European Convention on Human Rights, and in this context, Art 2, safeguarding the right to life may well be relevant. In particular, the person who suffers avoidable injury through the doctor's non-assistance might argue that the law's failure to impose liability upon the latter itself amounts to an infringement of his Art 2 right.[98]

11.2 Breach of Duty of Care

In England, in order to be liable in negligence, the healthcare professional must have breached his or her duty of care to the patient. The fact that A owes a duty of care to B, and that B suffers injury while under A's care, does not necessarily mean that A is liable in negligence to B or that B can win compensation (a sum of money for damage incurred) from A. If, for example, the risk of the harm suffered by B is inherent to the treatment, and B has provided valid consent to it, A is probably not liable in negligence (provided that the doctor has fulfilled his or her duty to inform adequately the patient, and that the patient's consent is valid—see earlier in this chapter).

In England the duty of care is quantified and qualified in terms of a *standard* that is reasonable to expect of a responsible professional. This has been established following a number of legal cases.[99] These cases draw general conclusions as to when professionals (not only medical professionals) can be said to have acted substandardly or to be responsible for harm to others (patients or clients). One of the most important of these cases is probably the one concerning Mr. Bolam (hence the term 'Bolam test').[100] This was mentioned earlier in this chapter while discussing the notion of best interests. The case, briefly, went as follows. In 1954, John Bolam was admitted to a psychiatric ward. He was diagnosed with depression. It was decided that he should be treated with electroconvulsive therapy (ECT). Nowadays, ECT is administered for severe depression under a general anaesthetic and with use of a muscle relaxant. In 1954, the use of a muscle relaxant was not as established as it is today. It was known, however, that the use of ECT without muscle relaxants might cause spasms, which may result in torn muscles and fractured bones. In the psychiatric ward where Bolam was admitted, the policy was not to administer muscle relaxants. The doctor in charge of Bolam, in accordance with the hospital policy, did not provide muscle relaxants, and Bolam ended up with a fractured hip. Bolam claimed compensation for negligence. But the treating doctors were not held negligent, because, it was argued, the doctors acted in accordance with a practice accepted as proper by a body of medics skilled in that particular treatment at the time. This case set up a legal precedent for breach of duty—the *Bolam* test: the standard of skill and care expected of a professional (including doctors) will be that of a skilled professional specialising in that particular field. This also means that, in case of litigation, it is virtually inevitable that the courts would require expert evidence, that is, that they would ask other professionals specialising in that particular field whether they would have done what the defendant did in the given circumstances. In principle, the *Bolam* test indicates that the defendant is not being careless and, hence, not negligent if skilled and competent professionals would have done the same in the given circumstances, even if harm to the patient has occurred and even if a different body of opinion exists which would take a contrary view. As established in the *Bolam* case, the professional is not guilty of negligence if s/he acted "in accordance with a practice accepted as proper by a responsible body of medical men skilled in that particular area".[101]

A later case, *Bolitho*,[102] also mentioned earlier, tempered the norm established in *Bolam*. The obvious worry arising from *Bolam* was that a professional would not be held negligent, insofar as expert witnesses were found who would act similarly to the defendant, regardless of whether or not the action taken was reasonable and responsible. In *Bolitho* the courts established that the professional's opinion also needs to be reasonable or responsible, and that it must withstand logical scrutiny.[103] This, of course, only relates to cases in which the professional has a duty of care towards the patient. The next element of negligence is causation.

11.3   Causation

Causation is probably the hardest element to prove in a claim in negligence. The onus of proof (balance of probabilities) generally lays on the patient.

The patient must prove that "if the defendant had behaved properly (ie not been in breach), the claimant would not have suffered the injury: this is known as the 'but for test'".[104] Where causal connection is absent or cannot be proven, a breach of standards of care does not amount to negligence. The breach of duty must be the cause of harm; there must be an unbroken chain of causation. For example, in the healthcare context, in *Barnett v. Chelsea and Kensington Hospital Management*,[105] three night watchmen went to a casualty department, complaining of abdominal pain after drinking tea. The doctor failed to examine them, advising that they see their own GP. One of the three men died soon after leaving the hospital. It was then found that the cause of death was arsenic poisoning. The case was brought to court, and the doctor was found to have breached his duty of care. However, expert evidence showed that, even if the doctor had fulfilled his duty of care, the watchman would have died anyway. Death, thus, was not imputable to a breach of duty of care, and consequently the doctor was not found negligent, although he was in breach of his duty of care because the claim failed on causation.[106] Having to prove that it is the doctor's breach to have caused the injury or harm of which the patient complains can "make things very awkward for claimants", especially "in cases where medical opinion is divided as to whether such conduct accorded with responsible medical practice or not".[107] An additional difficulty is represented by the fact that proving causation involves a counterfactual reasoning: what would have happened if the defendant had properly performed his or her duty. This makes causation difficult to prove because, as Stauch, Wheat, and Tingle note:

> The claimant—at the time of the doctor's breach—is normally already at risk of suffering an adverse outcome: in the context of a non-treatment case as here, the risk is posed by the illness that led him to seek the doctor's assistance. Here, it is always open to the doctor to argue that the patient's injury was due to the progress of the illness, which, even with all due medical care, could not have been arrested; if that is the case, the risk posed by the doctor's faulty non-treatment will remain just that—it will not have materialised in the sense of playing a necessary part in (ie causing) the harm.[108]

11.4 Foreseeability

The final requisite for negligence to occur is the foreseeability of the consequences (or harm incurred). In general, if the consequences of which the claimant complains were not reasonably foreseeable by the doctor, a claim of negligence is unlikely to succeed. It could be asked whether healthcare professionals could be held partly responsible for harm that is foreseeable, but which occurs outside the therapeutic relationship. For example, would a doctor be responsible if he insists that the applicant does not need hormonal treatment, and the applicant seeks such treatment via illegal routes and suffers harm following this? Would the doctor be responsible if, for example, this applicant contracted a disease from using unsterile needles? Would the doctor be responsible for the poor physical outcome of injecting hormones at unregulated doses or for the harm of having to undertake surgery, such as a mastectomy, which could have been avoided with early treatment?

It is difficult to give a straight answer to these questions, as it would depend on the circumstances of the case. It would be left to the judges to decide. In principle, a person can be held responsible for creating a source of danger even if s/he does not directly cause harm.[109] In spite of this, and in spite of best interests now encompassing more than purely clinical issues, for the reasons explained, a claim in negligence for *not receiving* treatment for gender dysphoria is perhaps unlikely to succeed, at least in England. Probably there would be a better chance in cases in which a patient was admitted but provided with medications in dosages and modalities that were not beneficial to the patient (a similar case has been discussed in Chapter 5). However, the four components of negligence would have to be proven in all cases.

A patient who is refused medical care is more likely to obtain treatment by requesting judicial review or by applying to a court (as Alex's aunt did in Australia) rather than by attempting to prove negligence. Judicial review is a process by which a High Court reviews a decision made by a public body—which may be a court, a tribunal, or another organisation.

> Judicial review allows individuals, businesses, and other groups to challenge the lawfulness of decisions made by Ministers, Government Departments, local authorities and other public bodies. The main grounds of review are that the decision maker has acted outside the scope of its statutory powers, that the decision was made using an unfair procedure, or that the decision was an unreasonable one. The Human Rights Act 1998 created an additional ground, making it unlawful for public bodies to act in a way incompatible with Convention rights.[110]

In the UK there is no known case of a patient applying to the courts or for judicial review to obtain early treatment for gender dysphoria. Patients' support groups suggest that the costs and time associated with such applications mean that people are better off travelling abroad, where they can receive privately paid treatment.[111]

11.5   Later Regret

Could doctors be exposed in allegations for malpractice if a patient complained about the therapy at a later stage? It would be difficult to accuse a doctor in malpractice for having administered treatment that is supported by a significant body of clinical literature and published research, that is, in line with international established guidelines, and to which the patient has given valid consent. A doctor can lawfully offer treatment provided that:

1. Treatment appears in the best interests of the applicant.
2. The treatment is offered according to the modalities suggested by well established guidelines, either national or international (see Chapter 5).
3. The treatment is supported by an authoritative body of medical opinion, as demonstrated by published research.
4. The treatment appears reasonable and withstands logical analysis and is responsibly given.
5. Valid consent is obtained (for more details on valid consent, see earlier in this chapter).
6. The clinician has the competencies and credentials to provide treatment, as explained, for example, in WPATH's *Standards of Care*.[112]

Even if a patient later regrets having commenced treatment, a claim against the treating doctors would be unlikely to succeed in these circumstances, provided that the risks (including the 'risk' of later regret) are dutifully explained.

One further question: can a doctor outside an established clinic lawfully provide medical treatment to transgender minors? In any one country, generally there is at the most one clinic that specialises in treatment of minors with gender dysphoria. If a sufferer is refused care by the clinic and obtained a referral to another paediatric endocrinologist, this other doctor, even if operating outside the 'main' clinic, could in principle offer treatment, provided that s/he satisfies the points just outlined. In the 2011 version of the *Standards of Care*, WPATH specifies what credentials and competencies doctors should have in order to be deemed suitable to treat transgender patients.[113] Although the multisciplinary aspects of the care for the transsexual are noted, there is no strict norm stated by WPATH advising that transgenders must solely be treated in a specialised clinic and by a team of specialists. Similarly, the Endocrine Society stresses that it would be ideal to have a multidisciplinary team treating the transgender patient, but recognises that this is not always possible, and it advises therefore that clinicians understand the contribution of various disciplines and communicate throughout the process.[114] WPATH also insists on the flexible nature of the guidelines, which must be adapted by health professionals to the needs of the individual patients: harm reduction is contemplated among the legitimate goals of health professionals. As we saw in Chapter 5, WPATH recognises that whereas the goal of therapy should be for the individual to find a gender role that is comfortable for them, the methods are likely to differ case by case. Medical intervention may be necessary for many people, but hormones and surgery "are just two of many options available to assist people with achieving comfort with self and identity".[115] It may be deducted that whereas the guidelines overall stress the multidisciplinary nature of gender identity treatment, and thus, whereas ideally a patient should be treated by a team of specialists, it is not against good clinical practice to offer treatment to individual patients, if the guidelines are followed and if individual health professionals have the credentials and competencies carefully outlined in the *Standards of Care*.

One final question is whether it would still be lawful to offer that treatment if in the established clinic that treatment is provided within a research study, as it happens in the UK. If the 'monitoring' (the research) is also meant to protect the individual patient from the yet unknown potential risks of treatment, it could be argued that other doctors could not provide that treatment unless they can monitor the effects of medications in a similar way, that is, unless they can also set up a research study and treat the patient also as a research participant. This raises an interesting question in law. How such a case would be treated by the courts or by the GMC in the UK is difficult to predict. It must, however, be mentioned that early treatment for gender dysphoria is *therapy* according to the wider international clinical community. As stated earlier, there is no suggestion in any of the main guidelines that this treatment ought to be provided exclusively within a research study. It may be good to systematically study the long term effects of this treatment, but this choice should not in principle cloud the fact that this is medical treatment whose main purpose is to benefit the individual patient, and that as such should be offered, even where the effects of medications are monitored in the long term. It could be argued that a patient who is unwilling, for whatever reason, to enter a research study should not, in principle, be denied the needed medical treatment.

12   CONCLUSIONS

The clinical encounter between trans minors and doctors is rich in legal complexities. This chapter does not do justice to all legal issues that could be relevant to our case. However, I have tried to examine the main concerns that doctors or patients could have. I have focused on English law, and where possible I have indicated the principles that may operate in different legislations. We have seen that minors can usually be treated in their best interests and that, in some circumstances, they can consent. The doctor has an obligation to provide the relevant information to the patient, including information relating to the possible unpredictable risks of the treatment sought. Where the treatment appears experimental in some ways and to some extent, due to its innovative nature, it will be prudent to gather the consent of the parents or those with parental responsibility. They should be involved anyway wherever possible, given that treatment for gender dysphoria encompasses the family and the wider social circle in a significant way, and having support may be essential to the individual patient.

Whereas doctors may be understandably wary of providing treatment with uncertain outcomes to children, provided that they operate in a responsible, reasonable manner, in accordance with established medical opinion, supported by published research and authoritative guidelines of clinical practice, they should be able to intervene in the best interests of the minor.

KEY POINTS

- Trans children and adolescents can be lawfully treated in their best interests.
- In cases of doubt, the doctors can seek assistance of the courts in England.
- Trans children and adolescents do not necessarily lack capacity to consent to treatment or to participate in the therapeutic relationship.
- The views of trans children and adolescents should be given adequate weight in the clinical relationship.
- Because of the experimental nature of early treatment, it is more prudent to always request parents' participation and consent to early treatment.
- If treatment is refused, a claim in negligence is unlikely to succeed in England, and judicial review can be requested.
- Parents who feel they have been unjustly refused treatment can apply for judicial review or to the courts.

8 Epistemological Issues Relating to Transgenderism[1]

*"We are not Christians"—they say—and Christ stopped at Eboli...
and the proverbial sentence that I have so many times heard [. . .] we
are not Christians, we are not men, but beasts, or less then beasts,
fruschi, frusculicchi, who live their diabolic or angelic life, because
we must instead be subjected to the world of the Christians, who
are beyond the horizon, and we have to bear their weight and their
comparison.*

(Carlo Levi, Cristo si è fermato ad Eboli)[2]

1 INTRODUCTION

We are in Lucania, in the south of Italy. Lucania (now called Basilicata)
is historically one of the poorest and most forgotten areas of Italy. Carlo
Levi, a Jewish doctor from Turin, is confined here in 1935. He discovers
a desolated land. Women are witches, and men are farmers who leave at
dark to reach the fields, two- to four-hour walk from town, and get back at
sunset, with no awareness, "like a tide".[3] The villages are fragile, built in
malarious bricks of clay, prone to disaster and collapse. In the baleful heat
of the Lucanian summer, Levi begins to understand that there is a parallel
dimension to the one he had known, a third way of being human.

In 1945 Levi publishes *Christ Stopped at Eboli*. In the language of the
southern Italians, being a Christian simply means *being a man*. As the epi-
graph to the chapter illustrates, the people at the time did not consider
themselves to be *human*, because they were outside the borders of humankind. People from Lucania, albeit formally Italian, do not have political
conscience: they are neither citizens nor contesters, neither fascists nor partisans, neither conationals nor enemies, they are just *beyond the state*. They
are not *Christians*, they are *frusculicchi*: they live in a third unrecognised
dimension; they are inhabitants of no man's land.

This is how the 'third sex' is sometimes described: as a no man's land.[4]
The very word 'trans-sexual', as we saw earlier in this book, was only
coined recently, whereas the phenomenon of crossing genders has, of course,
always been a part of human histories in virtually all cultures (although the
social—and legal—response to it has been markedly varied). We have also
seen that the term that is supposed to best capture the condition of gender
minorities is widely disputed: any term seems to cloud the rich diversity in
which gender can develop (see Chapter 1).

The history of transsexualism raises many important sociological and ethical issues relating to the legitimisation of minorities, to the sensibility of the very concepts of sex and gender used in medicine and at law, and to many others. In this chapter I discuss some fundamental epistemological issues around gender identity development as, unless there are sound reasons to consider gender variance as a mental illness, its inclusion in psychiatric diagnostic manuals risks being not only a conceptual mistake, but also a moral wrong done to those affected.

In January 2010 the Council of Europe stressed that considering gender variance as a mental illness may contradict the statement, as contained in the Universal Declaration of Human Rights, that "all human beings are born free and equal in dignity and rights",[5] and on 23 June 2011 the council launched the report *Combating Discrimination on Grounds of Sexual Orientation or Gender Identity—Council of Europe Standards*, stressing the need to protect the human rights of lesbian, gay, bisexual, and transgender people across Europe. Just before then, on 17 June 2011, the United Nations Human Rights Council adopted a resolution which expresses concerns about violence and discrimination against people because of their sex and gender orientation.[6] The World Professional Association for Transgender Health (WPATH) released a statement in May 2010 "urging the de-psychopathologization of gender conformity worldwide [. . .] the expression of gender characteristics, including identities, that are not stereotypically associated with one's assigned sex at birth is a common and culturally-diverse human phenomenon [that] should not be judged as inherently pathological or negative".[7] Gender identity is one of the most important, intimate, and private aspects of who we are. Gender identity like sexual orientation, concerns nobody else except for the person him/herself.[8] Considering gender diversity as a mental disorder may be, to use Marcuse's epithet, a form of "repressive tolerance".[9]

2   WHY 'GID' IS CONSIDERED A MENTAL ILLNESS

As we saw in Chapter 4, Gender Identity Disorder (GID) is classified as a psychiatric disorder. It is worth repeating here what the diagnostic criteria for GID are in the DSM-IV (the ICD has similar criteria—see Chapter 4):

- There is evidence of strong and persistent cross-gender identification.
- This cross-gender identification must not merely be a desire for any perceived cultural advantages of being the other sex.
- There must also be evidence of persistent discomfort about one's assigned sex or a sense of inappropriateness in the gender role of that sex.
- The individual must not have a concurrent physical intersex condition.
- There must be evidence of clinically significant distress or impairment in social, occupational, or other important areas of functioning.[10]

Whereas the psychiatric diagnosis has apparent advantages (some of these will be discussed later in this chapter), it also has potential psychological and social adverse implications.[11] It is therefore important to assess whether gender variance is appropriately conceptualised as a mental disorder, and, if not, what the normative implications of this are.

I consider in particular three main epistemological reasons for enclosing gender variance among mental disorders:

- The first is that gender variance is associated with extreme psychological/emotional distress and with impairment in social and occupational or other important areas of functioning (see Section 2).[12]
- The second is that no single somatic cause or set of causes has been found, which may explain the discomfort (see Section 3)—the implication being that thus the condition must be psychological in nature.
- The third is that gender variance is perhaps not a *mental* disorder, but is nonetheless a disorder or illness as it is a marked deviance from a norm, where the norm in this case is defined in terms of "normal species functioning" (see Section 4).[13]

I select these arguments because they form a part of the main assumptions implicitly or explicitly accepted by a part of the scholarly literature on gender variance (see the following).

It should be noted that I am not in this way proposing a definition of mental illness, nor am I evaluating whether any of these epistemological reasons is a sufficient or a necessary condition to consider any given human experience as a mental illness. Moreover, for the purposes of this chapter, I assume that there is such a thing as a mental illness/mental disorder, without discussing the epistemological issues relating to these very notions.[14] I rely on the characterisation of mental disorder proposed, for example, by the DSM.[15] Central to it is the presence of a psychological or behavioural pattern associated with distress, which is not a part of normal development or culture,[16] and which involves "clinically significant distress or impairment in social, occupational, or other important areas of functioning" (the so called clinical significance criterion).[17] It is worth stressing, however, that many have contested that there is such a thing as a 'mental' illness, and it is only for the purposes of this argument that it is presumed in this chapter that the notion has any meaning at all.

3   GENDER MINORITIES, SUFFERING, AND PSYCHOSOCIAL FUNCTIONING

Gender variance is invariably connected with suffering and it alters social adjustment and functioning: typically the individual and the significant others are profoundly affected by the discovery that gender identification is not the one they expected.[18] Gender variance also alters the person's ability to function socially and is often associated with poor psychological and social outcome especially when proper medical care is not provided in a timely manner.[19]

Contrary to what may appear, these are not appropriate grounds for conceptualising gender variance as a mental disorder, for at least two reasons.

First, many conditions are associated with suffering and significant impairments in the life of the individual and the family. Breaking up, bereavement, and many other events may have similar consequences, but are not for that reason *mental illnesses*. Either it is accepted that, in fairness, many more conditions should be included in psychiatric manuals or it must be accepted that that ground may be shaky.

One may object that perhaps suffering and impairment in psychosocial functioning are not *per se* grounds to consider a condition as a psychiatric condition. However, the presence of distress and the adverse psychosocial sequelae may perhaps be *an indication of* a mental disorder, depending on circumstances and scales of the problem. For example, bereavement may cause extreme distress and psychosocial dysfunction. But if I am unable to work and function socially because my cat died a year ago, my bereavement may be an indication of a disorder of mind, even if, *per se*, bereavement is not a mental disorder.

On this ground, gender variance should be regarded as a mental disorder depending on the modality in which the individual reacts to his or her gender identification. This, apparently, seems to be what happens in clinical practice: if an individual has *some kind of* gender dysphoria, s/he is not for that reason diagnosed as having a mental disorder. The diagnosis is only attached to severe, persistent discomfort associated with negative psychosocial sequelae.

However, this objection is question begging: persistent and severe gender dysphoria is still regarded as a mental disorder, and this is precisely what needs to be justified. The problem, from a conceptual point of view, is why me not feeling the congruence between my body and my identity is regarded as psychopathological; of course, to respond that having a mild discomfort is not psychopathological does not answer the question.

Second, and perhaps more importantly, distress may be an *adequate* response to adversities. The example of bereavement fits well in this context. If I am no longer able to work and function in the same way I used to, because my son, rather than my cat, has died, my response may be adequate to the circumstances. What is *an adequate* response to events is, of course, open to debate, and there are significant grey areas of uncertainty. Some may say, for example, that even if I lose my child at some point in the future I should be able to 'recover' and resume a seemingly 'normal' life; others may argue that this would be impossible and that I could never be expected to live as normal in those circumstances; others may argue that perhaps the age of the child may make a difference: should I lose my newborn baby the trauma may not be as profound as losing my ten-year-old son . . . and so on . . . Evaluating people's responses to adverse events obviously encounters endless conceptual and ethical problems. What this shows, however, is important and relevant to the understanding of what happens to gender minorities: it is not distress or psychosocial dysfunction *per se* that reveal the existence of a problem in someone's emotional or psychological life. A much larger perspective must be adopted in order to evaluate the adequacy of someone's distress as a response to any particular event in any given context.

In the case of gender minorities, distress may be an understandable (and perhaps adequate) response to adverse social variables and to a hostile environment. If my five-year-old boy insists on buying pink trainers with sparkles and consequently he is ridiculed at school by his peers, his upset and secrecy would be appropriate responses to the circumstances. Of course, we would all expect children to mix up and enjoy their childhood and be happy. But we know that stereotypes (sometimes rigidly internalised by children) may prevent acceptance of diversity. Thus the 'psychosocial dysfunction' rather than being the indication of an intrapsychic problem, may reveal a problem in the social context in which the individual happens to live. In fact, the ill psychosocial adjustment typically associated with gender variance seems to be, to a significant extent, a function of societal inability to embrace gender differences as normal (and nonpathological) and treat them as such (see earlier in this book). The Council of Europe has emphasised with great concern the high degrees of discrimination, abuse, and violence to which LGBTs are subjected.[20] Even in the absence of physical or verbal abuse, the marginalisation of the gender minority is apparent: marriage, employment, and many legal rights are often a function of 'gender'.[21] Birth itself is marked by gender predictions and those who do not fit a mainstream gender divide are left in a legal and social vacuum.[22]

Some people with gender dysphoria narrate the grief associated with having to continually pretend to be someone they are not, being scared of being caught or uncovered. They tell of secretly sneaking into their sibling's room to wear their clothes and about the relief of those minutes in which one could finally pretend to be him/herself. People are secretive and ashamed about how they feel. Being frightened of the response they might get, some people hide for many years and live in the grief of a continued lie to all others, often including their parents, partners, and children (see Chapter 4 for narrations). The intra-psychic suffering, thus, is inextricably intertwined with the moral and cultural imperatives accepted or internalised by the society in which the sufferer happens to live.

To describe gender minorities as suffering from a mental disorder because they lack serene psychosocial adjustment is to condemn them to a double jeopardy: they do not have the possibility of serene psychological and social adjustment because the existence of a normal, nonpathological 'different' way of being is not accommodated, and then they are regarded as mentally ill because they have not adjusted well.

4   GENDER DYSPHORIA HAS NO CAUSE

The hypothesis that gender variance may be caused by some physical disorder has attracted much attention in scientific settings: finding a somatic cause of gender dysphoria would have, at least apparently, a number of advantages. It would allow removal of GID from psychiatric manuals and inclusion in, for example, endocrinological manuals (with the consequent reduction of stigma associated with the psychiatric diagnosis). At the same time, it would apparently strengthen people's entitlement to publicly funded medical treatment or to reimbursement under insurance schemes.

The first candidates for the search for 'natural error' have been genes and chromosomes. Extensive research has been performed on the relationship between gender variance and endocrinological disorders such as disorders or sex development (DSDs) or intersex conditions. These conditions affect the development of primary and secondary sex characteristics. As mentioned earlier in the book, research has shown that, although there is a higher prevalence of gender variance amongst people with DSDs than in the 'normal' population, DSDs are not always associated with gender variance.[23] Gender variance is a different condition and often unrelated to DSDs, and DSDs are not the cause of gender variance.[24]

It could be argued that in absence of a physiological explanation to gender variance, the condition must be psychological in nature. This is an argument that, implicitly or explicitly, recurs both in common discourse and in the literature on gender dysphoria.[25] As Raymond also points out, the term *psychiatric syndrome*, used to refer to the condition, "probably indicates that transsexualism [is not considered] to be of biological origin".[26]

There are a number of flaws in these types of assertions.

- First, *prima facie*, the absence of a somatic cause is arguably an indication that there is no pathology rather than that there is psychopathology,[27] even in the presence of distress.
- Second, the very notion of mental illness is contentious, and, if used to denote situations of distress that are unexplained by somatic factors, risks becoming the collection box of experiences and behaviours that are difficult to understand. This could have wider implications: for example, the psychiatric diagnosis may become an instrument of social control,[28] and it may detract attention from the relational or social causes of distress.
- Third, this argument implies that body and mind are two ontologically separate entities. Gilbert Ryle spoke about this 'Cartesian' belief

as *a myth, a dogma*,[29] which is as largely accepted as it is philosophi-
cally or scientifically unproven.[30]

- Fourth, the fact that the causes of gender variance are unknown does
  not mean that they do not exist. It is possible that research development will identify some somatic causes for gender variance, and that
  gender identity development will be understood better at some point.

Finally, there is an important point to note. The causes of atypical gender
identification are unknown. Likewise, the causes of *typical gender identification* also are. The hypothesis that gender develops 'quite naturally' based
on our genetic and chromosomal endowment is a mistake. The basic biological facts (determination of sex) are not straightforward (see also Chapters 2 and 3).[31] Even considering the basic biological facts, there is no clear
'order' to which one may refer in order to determine the 'disorder'.

The construction of gender, the adoption of gender roles, and the adaptation to gender expectations are determined by biological and social forces,
which interact in a somewhat mysterious way to shape who each of us is.
There are various theories of gender development, as discussed earlier. Yet,
ultimately, how genes, social stressors, and historical and cultural variables
interact to make each of us into the 'gendered' individuals we are is unknown.
How gender identity develops is an open question both in 'atypical' and in
'typical' cases, as discussed in Chapter 3. This seems to imply that there is no
clear set of biological or social markers to which one could cling to determine
which gender developments are 'normal' and which are 'pathological'.

The belief that, in nature, there are men and women, or that those who
do not fit the divide are *disordered*, is thus a superstition, and it is no less of
a superstition than the belief that there are *frusculicchi* or that your future
is written in the lines of your hand.

The claim that some types of gender development are *disordered*, thus,
seems to mean that they *deviate* from what happens to the majority of
people. I will deal with this argument in the next section.

5   GENDER AS VARIATION FROM
NORMAL SPECIES FUNCTIONING

It could be argued that maybe gender development is not yet understood;
however, without a doubt in the vast majority of cases gender development
does not cause the distress we see in children with atypical gender. Most
people grow in the gender assigned to them at birth, and do so quite com-
fortably. If some people do not develop in a similar way, then this fact in
itself may be an indication that there is pathology. Add to this the fact that
gender dysphoria is always marked by great confusion and distress, then
one may reasonably conclude that there must be some kind of pathology,
even if the aetiology is unknown.

Of all the arguments examined so far, this is the most problematic, both from a conceptual and from an ethical point of view. The vexed question of 'what is a disability' has challenged philosophers and medical ethicists for some time. Indeed, sometimes 'illness' has been defined in terms of deviation from "normal species functioning".[32] I will not repeat here the controversies surrounding the notions of disorder/illness/disability.[33] What is important to note is that an illness, and thus also a *mental illness*, cannot simply be defined in terms of *variation from what happens in the vast majority of cases* (even if it is a variation associated with great distress). The vast majority of people are right-handed, and yet being left-handed is not pathology. The majority of adults in Western countries perhaps are short-sighted, and yet having twenty-twenty vision is not for that reason an illness.

Being a part of a numerical difference is no indication of illness. To consider gender, which is a form of private and intimate difference, as 'mental illness' is not real acceptance of the difference as a fully legitimate fact, but willingness to endure it, on the condition that it is marked out as 'anomalous' and 'sick'. "This sort of tolerance" wrote Marcuse, is "repressive tolerance"; it "strengthens the tyranny of the majority".[34]

"Majorities", said the poet De André, "have the bad habit to look over their shoulders, and to count, and to say 'we are six hundred millions, we are one billion and two hundred millions', and, taking advantage of being so numerous, they think they are able to, they are entitled to disturb, to humiliate, the minorities".[35]

There are, of course, various ways to humiliate: verbal and physical abuse are only two of these. To condemn a minority to the stigma of mental illness with no sound reason is another way. It is true that distress is associated with gender variance: however, this distress is significantly a function of societal inability to embrace gender differences as normal, and in societies where the gender divide is not as marked, transsexuals suffer less.[36] The stigma of the psychiatric diagnosis marks out this difference as a disorder, and thus risks reinforcing some of the very causes of distress.

6 PRAGMATIC REASONS TO RETAIN THE PSYCHIATRIC DIAGNOSIS

There may be other important reasons, which are not epistemological, for retaining the formal diagnosis of GID. For example, it has been argued that a formal diagnosis encourages research development,[37] that it helps make more reliable predictions and therefore avoid treating false positives: for instance, Wallien and Cohen-Kettenis suggest that children who meet the complete DSM-IV criteria for GID are more likely to be persisters.[38] Moreover, the psychiatric diagnosis provides a sort of (possibly reassuring) 'explanation' for seemingly inexplicable experiences; it can protect both sufferer and the significant others from feelings of guilt and blame, which are often associated with 'abnormal' behaviours; perhaps more importantly, a formal diagnosis might facilitate access to NHS treatment or insurance coverage.

These reasons do not relate to *how we may understand gender variance*, or any other human experience, and in this sense are not epistemological in nature. They have to do with the *practical consequences* that retaining the diagnosis has for the people concerned, for their families, for the medical profession, and for society at large, but are not for this less important: if retaining the psychiatric diagnosis was highly likely to promote and protect people's welfare, this would provide a strong *prima facie* reason in its favour.

However these pragmatic reasons are not straightforward.

6.1   The Relationship between Diagnosis and Treatment

With regard to access to treatment, medical treatment for gender variance is complex and long lasting (see Chapter 5). One worry may be that removal of GID from psychiatric manuals could affect the sufferers' right to access medical treatment or to funded treatment. However, this is not necessarily the case. In the United Kingdom, for example, Primary Care Trusts (PCTs) make decisions on the matter depending on budget. In May 2010 breast surgery was refused to a transgender with the argument that this is 'cosmetic surgery'.[39] According to the Gender Research and Education Society 2009 Report,[40] the NHS may fund the following treatment for male to female trans:

i. orchidectomy—removal of testicles
ii. penectomy
iii. vaginoplasty
iv. clitoroplasy
v. labioplasty
vi. hair removal—donor site

Mammoplasty (breast enlargement) thyroid chondroplasty (reduction of the Adam's apple), facial feminising (like reshaping of the nose and chin), body reshaping, cricothyroid approximation and other vocal surgery to raise the pitch of the voice, hair removal of the face and body, and hair transplant (to mitigate male baldness) are not typically funded publicly.

For female to male trans, the following are usually funded by the NHS:

i. mastectomy
ii. hysterectomy
iii. vaginectomy
iv. salpingo-oohrectomy—removal of the fallopian tubes and ovaries

   v. metoidioplasy—creation of micro-penis using the clitoris
  vi. phalloplasty—creation of penis, with or without the urethra
 vii. urethroplasty—creation of urethra within the penis
viii. scrotoplasty—creation of scrotum
  ix. placement of testicular prostheses

Not included are penile prosthesis, that is, an implant that makes erection possible, and hair removal (donor site). It is clear that the list of funded treatment is not inclusive of all procedures that are necessary to confirm one's gender. Therefore, there is a doubt that the psychiatric diagnosis can grant publicly funded healthcare interventions. Things may be even trickier in other countries, where the psychiatric diagnosis can become a boomerang. In the US, for example, insurance companies generally offer coverage only for 'psychiatric' treatment for diagnosed mental illnesses. Therefore, they may subsidise psychotropic drugs for depression and anxiety that may be associated with GID, but hormonal treatments and surgery, which may be needed by people with gender variance, might be excluded from insurance coverage.[41] Therefore, the psychiatric diagnosis may be a boomerang: it may not help sufferers to obtain the medical care they may need, and it may instead reduce their chance to obtain the needed publicly funded treatment.

It should also be noted that, if the concern is access to medical treatment, there are alternatives to the psychiatric diagnosis. For example, in view of the similarities experienced by sufferers and of the significant numbers of people affected, one possibility would be to regard the condition as a *syndrome*. A syndrome is a cluster of experiences and phenomena that "run together",[42] that are seen in association, whose aetiology is often unknown. These are not psychiatric conditions, and are not even regarded as illnesses, strictly speaking.

Even if whatever has to do with gender were demedicalised (like homosexuality and heterosexuality[43]), this should have no bearing upon access to treatment. Medical treatment should be offered based on need and prognosis, not based on nosology or on the classification of the sort of condition one has. I will discuss this at greater length in Chapter 9, but let us anticipate some considerations here.

6.1.1 Medical Treatment Should Only Be Offered for Illnesses

It could be argued that doctors have a moral obligation (*prima facie*) to treat people's *illnesses*, and that they do not have a comparable obligation to satisfy people's *preferences*. For example, it may be appropriate to offer breast reconstruction after a mastectomy due to cancer, but it is not equally appropriate to offer breast reconstruction if I want to look more feminine. You cannot claim a right to be cured if there is no illness to cure. Unless gender dysphoria is an illness, there is no right to medical treatment.

This argument rests on the idea that *medicine should only intervene to cure illnesses/disabilities*. As such, this argument is incomplete: it should be grounded on a somehow clear view of what constitutes an illness/disability, and what 'normality' is. As suggested before (and as discussed at great length in Chapter 3), it is not clear what 'normal' and 'abnormal' stand for here. More generally, the notions of illness, disorder, and disability (and other synonymous) are highly elusive, and there is no consensus as to how they should be understood or defined. In fact, arguably, the definition of 'illness' is not a primarily medical issue, but is primarily an ontological issue relating to what sort of entities humans are, and on axiological categories relating to what each of us believes a good life to be. Some have, for example, argued that deafness is not an illness but a desirable attribute.[44] This is because their axiological views differ from those of others: they believe that being unable to hear is a good thing, that it is better for some people overall to be deaf than to be hearing. For them, deafness is not an illness. This is just one illustration of how the definition of 'illness' cannot be provided by means of empirical observation: it is a matter of values, and of values over which consensus cannot necessarily be expected. The argument that medicine should only intervene to cure diseases or disabilities or illnesses thus is question begging, because one can ask what are the *illnesses or disabilities* which grant access to medical treatment, what is it that make some conditions *illnesses or disabilities*. Therefore, also the argument that people have a legitimate claim to medical treatment only insofar as they have a 'diagnosed' illness is at least incomplete.

There is another problem with the argument at stake here: it proposes an understanding of medicine that is too narrow.

6.1.2   *A Too Narrow Understanding of Medicine*

Intending medicine as an enterprise only aimed at curing diagnosed illnesses is too narrow a view of medicine, and one that is in contrast with the general understanding of what medicine is for. Many interventions are regarded as within the sphere of legitimate concerns of medicine, and yet do not repair illnesses, disabilities, or variations from normal functioning. On the contrary, often they *reverse* what appears to be 'normal functioning'. Earlier I made the examples of contraception and pain relief in labour. In both cases, there is no illness, no dysfunction, and what is happening is perfectly normal. Yet medical treatment is provided. The role of medicine is to improve people's quality of life, prevent harm, alleviate suffering (even suffering that is normally associated to a natural event). As also mentioned in Chapter 6, age related conditions are other examples of 'normal species functioning': it is 'normal' for postmenopausal woman to have reduced bone mineral density, yet medicine intervenes to 'treat' what is very normal species functioning, a very normal and spontaneous development, in order to prevent or alleviate suffering and improve quality of life. Another example is vasectomy: here a mutilation is performed, which reverts what appears perfectly 'normal' functioning in order to improve the person's quality of life. Countless examples similar to these could be provided.

In these and many other cases, the NHS or insurance companies pay for these interventions. Treatment for age related conditions is funded in the UK and reimbursed within many insurance schemes. Surgery for birth marks or 'bat ears' can be publicly funded in the UK. Insurance companies might pay for purely cosmetic surgery in cases of, for example, breasts disparities occurring at birth or as a result of other illnesses such as breast cancer.[45] In these cases, there might not be any 'medical' necessity to have additional surgery, and yet this is offered to alleviate psychological suffering and enhance quality of life.

This illustrates how often medicine intervenes with medical treatments and surgery when there is no diagnosed 'illness', and even to revert what is 'normal functioning'.

To return to gender dysphoria, it is thus unclear why removal of GID from diagnostic manuals in principle should affect people's entitlement to receive medical treatment, to public support under the NHS, or to insurance coverage under privately funded schemes.

6.1.3 Society Might Be Wrong, but This Is Not a Reason to Deny Medical Treatment

As we have also seen in Chapter 6, it could be objected that in cases where the condition is social in nature, that is, caused primarily or exclusively by social variables that are clearly identifiable, those social factors must be amended, rather than people's bodies. On this line, it could be objected to the arguments I proposed so far that in cases of pain relief or contraception or reversal of age related conditions there is an undesirable physical state that medicine can ameliorate. In the case of gender dysphoria, people instead appear to suffer primarily because of mistaken social norms and policies. If society is wrong, we should not mutilate people's bodies: we should endeavour to change society. We have seen in Chapter 6 that sometimes this argument has been stretched to the extreme of arguing that cross sex surgery reinforces the stereotypes that cause gender dysphoria, and is therefore immoral both for the individual and for society as a whole.

This argument is, however, also flawed. People often suffer due to a variety of reasons, which are at times inextricable. Some of these reasons are inherent to their condition, and some might be social or familial. This should have no bearing upon access to treatment. Indeed, this has no bearing in other cases of healthcare provision. I have already partly answered this objection in Chapter 6, but let us further this point.

For example, not wanting children is often a matter of social and cultural variables. Yet contraceptive treatment is provided and not denied based on the fact that it is sought for social reasons. In Chapter 6 I mentioned the example of fertility treatment: this can be provided, and is often publicly funded, regardless of how people came to be infertile or why they suffer being childless.

If we identify the social causes of people's unhappiness, we have a reason to try and amend these; yet medical treatment is typically provided not on the basis of whether or to what extent biological rather than social factors contribute to the applicant's request. Medical treatment is provided if people suffer and treatment can benefit them. If medical intervention appears to be in the applicant's interests, then in principle it should be offered.

To deny medical treatment to those who are in distress partly because of social reasons is to inflict a double jeopardy on them: they suffer a social wrong, and, in addition to this, medicine, which could help, fails to assist. Social intervention, such as changes in the law and in some social policies, as well as public education, may indeed all be necessary to fully address the legitimate needs of gender minorities; these, however, do not exclude the fact that medical intervention may also be necessary.

6.1.4   Treatment Should Be Given If It Is in the Person's Interests

Endocrinologists might feel unease in giving hormonal therapies, especially to young minors, when they have no hormonal defects or illnesses. However, medicine should serve the interests of patients, not of doctors.

Confining the role of medicine to the cure of illnesses not only meets with insurmountable conceptual problems relating to the definition of illness and normality; it also defies the scope of medicine. Medicine intervenes with medical therapies in cases in which there is not, strictly speaking, 'medical' necessity (see Chapter 6). If medical treatment is to be withdrawn in cases of gender issues because gender issues do not qualify as illnesses, or because they are to an important extent the result of social factors, many of other medical treatments should consistently be withdrawn as a matter of fairness.

6.1.5   Where Do We Draw the Line?

The absence of a diagnosis should not in principle have a bearing upon the right to access medical treatment and the right to public funds and insurance coverage. The test to assess whether treatment should be provided is whether people suffer and whether medical treatment could alleviate their suffering. If suffering can be alleviated, there is a *prima facie* moral reason to do so, and stringent moral reasons should be provided to justify denying beneficial medical interventions.

One could ask whether, on my account, the state or insurance companies should also provide for 'cosmetic' surgery: people could be in extreme distress because they dislike some of their body parts.[46] Or, more provocatively, one could ask whether on my account the state or insurance companies should also pay for recreational drugs to release the existential suffering of many young people on Friday nights.[47] I will return to these questions later in the book, but let's draw some indications of where this discourse may lead.

My account leaves a question open, of where society should draw the line between interventions that are needed *enough* to be provided and paid for and interventions that are somehow unwarranted or even unethical.

However, it is not 'my account' that does so: there are two broader questions. One is of how scarce resources should be distributed and what areas of healthcare should receive priority; the other is which medical requests can ethically be satisfied (regardless of who should pay for them). Examples of controversial medical interventions are blepharoplasty for Asian women; nose filing for black people; and skin bleaching and similar, derogatively called 'racial' surgical interventions. These issues are on the ethics agenda: however, these go beyond the discourse of gender identity. Medical intervention for gender minorities should certainly not be suspended until these broader issues are resolved.

The fundamental point here is that *if* GID were to be removed from the diagnostic manuals (as it should), *this would not mean, ipso facto, that medical treatment is unwarranted.* Where we should draw the line is certainly a problem over which we (philosophers, policymakers, and the general public) should reflect more. In the next chapter I will consider whether treatment for gender minorities should fall on one side of the line or on the other, and why this may be so. I will do so by considering the arguments for and against provision of care for gender variance.

On the other hand, it is a mistake to think that leaving GID in the psychiatric manuals grants access to treatment. As we have seen, the psychiatric diagnosis can be a boomerang: it might mean that hormonal and surgical interventions are excluded from coverage.

7 THE RELATIONSHIP BETWEEN DIAGNOSIS AND RESEARCH

With regard to research, research on gender development was carried out long before GID became a diagnostic category. We have seen in Chapter 3 how Bowlby and Bandura, for example, performed groundbreaking experimental studies already in the 1950s and 1960s. We have seen that former philosophers, such as Comte, Mill, and others, proposed theories relating to how gender should develop and what this should imply (see Chapter 2). This happened a long time before the nomenclature of GID even existed. There is no reason why research should be negatively affected by the removal of GID from the diagnostic manuals.

With regard to the reliability of predictions, if the DSM criteria prove helpful in order to frame strategies of intervention, then they should be used. This, however, does not imply that the psychiatric diagnosis must also be retained. In principle, the criteria could be used to assess whether and at what stage to begin medical treatment, without necessarily having to result in a psychiatric diagnosis.

With regard to the reassuring potential of the psychiatric diagnosis, indeed the person may not know or understand what is 'going wrong' with her/him, and being told that what is happening is a recognised disorder, with a name and clinical features that recur in a similar way in other people, may soothe anxiety.[48] But it is not clear why a sufferer and her/his family may not be equally reassured at hearing that gender variance is a normal way in which gender may develop; that there are many people similarly developing in an atypical way; that there is no pathology one should worry about; and that there is a wide range of medical, social, and lifestyle interventions that can help. It is unclear why a statement of normality should be less reassuring than a diagnosis of psychopathology.

Finally, there is something important to note with regard to the protection from guilt and blame. On the one hand, the diagnosis may help sufferers and families to tolerate what is happening; on the other hand, inclusion of GID in psychiatric manuals has not heralded greater social tolerance towards LBGTs. LBGTs remain one of the minorities most subjected to discrimination, abuse, violence, and murder.[49] The classification of gender variation as a mental illness can detract attention from the social forces that are responsible for the person's suffering, by reinforcing the prejudice that the problems of transsexuals are intra-psychic, that they lay principally within the affected person, and that they are not relational or cultural in any decisive way.

Thus, even considering the practical implications of retaining the psychiatric diagnosis, it is not clear that, on balance, this serves the interests of those affected.

8 CONCLUSIONS

Gender identity is a part of who we are, and it results from a mysterious interplay of biological and social forces. Both typical and atypical gender identification are poorly understood, and there are no clear biological markers of sex and gender development which could suggest that one way of being is healthy and another is pathological.

Accepting the existence of a variety of ways of being woman or man means looking beyond the stereotypical gender divide and accepting that all people "are born equal in dignity and right" regardless of their sex and gender orientation, and that their difference should not be regarded as deviance.[50]

In the absence of sound reasons, epistemological or otherwise, for retaining the psychiatric diagnosis of GID, the inclusion of gender variance amongst mental disorders, far from serving the interests of the people affected, may illustrate societal inability or unwillingness to recognise the full legitimacy of gender minorities and to consider atypical gender development as one of the different ways in which identity can be formed.

The people from Lucania taught Levi that those who are neither in the state nor outside the state are no less *human* than anyone else. They are not for that reason *frusculicchi*. In the case of Lucanian people, their difference related to the political state: they were neither in the regime nor against it. In our case, the difference relates to the state of being *a woman or a man*. If people go beyond the dichotomy of the classic gender divide and are a part of a gender minority, it does not mean they are for that reason *disordered*.

Regarding gender differences as mental disorders risks reinforcing the view that there are only two possible sound ways of being: male or female, a view that is problematic both from a scientific and from a conceptual and moral point of view. It also risks reinforcing discrimination against those who are a part of a minority, by perpetuating the view of atypical gender identification as a deviance. This contradicts the moral imperative that we all share to have equal concern and respect for all members of the human family,[51] regardless of arbitrary features and private aspects of personal identity, such as age, race, sexual orientation, or gender.

9   Should Gender Minorities Pay for Medical Treatment?

Ovla kon ascovi me gava palan ladi me gava palan bura ot croiuti.

I will follow this migration, I will follow this current of wings.

(F. De André and I. Fossati, 'Khorakhanè', 1996)[1]

1   INTRODUCTION[2]

The inclusion of transgenderism among mental illnesses is contentious.[3] As we saw in the previous chapter, the Council of Europe, in January 2010, also stressed the need for recasting transsexualism in terms of individual and private difference, rather than as a mental disorder (see also the 2011 documents quoted in the previous chapter). Some commentators have pointed out that the classification of Gender Identity Disorder (GID) among mental illnesses is by all means peculiar, in that the 'treatment' for it is at odds with any plausible conception of 'treatment': 'treatments' are supposed to eliminate or reduce the symptoms, whereas in the case of gender dysphoria, medical treatment proposes to alter the body in order to match the very belief that is regarded as the main manifestation of the alleged mental illness.[4] However, if GID were to be removed from diagnostic manuals, where would this leave people with gender dysphoria, in terms of access to medical care?[5] Should the state (or insurance companies) pay for medical treatment for gender issues?

2   METHODS

The methods used here are somewhat a departure from the typical methods of applied philosophy and from the methods used so far in this book. First, I ground this chapter on a thought experiment: the thought experiment is that GID is no longer officially regarded as pathology. Second, on this assumption, I construe two cases: one gestures towards the conclusion that, if it is accepted that gender issues are not pathology, then they should be treated in the same way as other types of body dissatisfaction: medical treatment should be negotiated by applicants and healthcare professionals, as in cases of 'cosmetic'[6] surgery; the transaction is a private matter and medical treatment should be paid for privately by the applicant. In the other line of argument it is claimed that gender issues are often not comparable, in normatively relevant ways, to other types of body dissatisfaction, and that it would be unethical to refuse funded medical treatment if that treatment is likely to prevent serious harm. Within each scenario, the arguments are explored with the classic methods of analytic philosophy: the morally relevant facts are identified, and the reasons for and against publicly funded or reimbursed care for gender issues are explored. Of course, it is possible to think about even more scenarios and arguments: those identified are possibly the most plausible that could be brought for and against publicly funded treatment for transgenderism.

In this way, I aim at illustrating some of the complexities relating to medical treatment for gender dysphoria and at showing how seemingly plausible arguments may prompt seemingly irreconcilable conclusions. I will not criticise each argument in turn, but, in running parallel scenarios, the arguments themselves will oppose one another, and the relative pitfalls of each contention will become apparent in the course of the chapter. I will in the end offer my resolution to the dilemma. I will argue that, in cases of gender identity issues, we have *prima facie* stringent moral reasons to offer funded medical treatment.

3 INSTRUCTIONS FOR CHAPTER USE

After reading the summary in Section 4, proceed to read scenario 1 and scenario 2. Both scenarios contain the same sections. When you move from one to the other, you may read the same arguments again, but they are presented in a way that leads to opposite conclusions. For reasons of simplicity, most references are only found in scenario 1. To make the reading somehow easier, I have labelled the sections in scenario 1 as S1.1, S.2, etc., and those in scenario 2 as S2.1, S2.2, and so on.

4 SLIDING DOORS: SUMMARY

Sliding Doors is a 1998 film directed by Peter Howitt, starring Gwyneth Paltrow. Here is a summary:

Helen is fired. She leaves her office to go back home. In the Underground her life is split. In one scenario, she gets on the train, and by chance she meets James, a charming man. But she gets home to find her partner in bed with his ex-girlfriend. She moves out, her life and career begin again, she meets James again, and in an accident, she dies. In the other scenario she misses the train, and, as she returns home later, she remains ignorant of the partner's affair. He does not work and she keeps supporting him with occasional jobs. . . eventually she meets the charming James. . . . . The film runs through double railways, in a paradoxical time overlap.

In the fiction proposed here we also have two scenarios. In both scenarios GID is removed from diagnostic manuals: the human right to be different is upheld; it is claimed that people should not be discriminated against, subjected to any form of abuse and violence for reasons relating to their sex and gender orientation; each individual should be free to explore and construct their identity, without for that reason having to pay the price of being called mentally ill, or the price of any other type of discrimination and abuse.

The difference between the two scenarios concerns what this personal freedom entails, and here the chapter splits. . . .

SLIDING DOORS

SCENARIO 1

S1.1   Felines, Star Treks, and Other Varieties: Should Doctors Do This?

People may be unhappy with some body parts: the fact itself is of no surprise. But sometimes, dissatisfaction may be extreme. Some people would rather not be human. The woman known as the 'Cat Woman' or the 'Cat Lady' underwent several interventions of facial surgery to look like a cat. She has had surgery on her eyes, which have been pulled up and back; she has had several silicone injections to her lips, cheeks, and chin, and a facelift in order for her face to look feline. The fiction *Star Trek* prompted another fashion: the application of silicon to look like the characters of the film. Various trends include 'sacrification' (skin cutting or marking), ear cutting and reshaping (generally to produce appearance similar to the elves), tongue splitting (to replicate the snake's tongue), and others.[7] People, of course, also seek what may appear to be more moderate interventions. For example, a growing number of Asian women seek blepharoplasty,[8] and an increasing number of black women seek surgery to look more Caucasian.[9] Whereas these types of medical interventions might seem less extreme than the ones reported before, they give rise to perhaps more acute ethical dilemmas, as they are based on 'suspect'[10] norms of social acceptability. In some cases, these norms are inherently racist and are more worrying to the extent that they are internalised by the person belonging to the discriminated group. It could be argued that the medical profession, by providing medical treatment to people seeking 'racial' surgery,[11] somehow contributes to the idea that, in order to be acceptable, a person must conform to a stated normative aesthetic standard, which is arguably racist.

Let's see what this all has to do with transsexualism and access to medical treatment.

S1.2   The Case of Gender Identity

Ethically, those interventions that seek to amend ethnic features, as well as many so called 'cosmetic' types of surgery, such as breast implants, liposuction, and so on, may be even more problematic than a (more unconventional and perhaps more 'autonomous' or personal) preference to look like Mr. Spock. They in fact appear to induce people to conform to (or reveal the way in which people internalise) stated standards of social acceptability, which are suspect or even openly racist.

(continued)

SCENARIO 1 (continued)

Not dissimilarly to many of those seeking 'cosmetic' and 'racial' surgery, people with gender dysphoria also appear to suffer because of 'suspect' norms of social acceptability. In many Western societies it is assumed that people should be either men or women. The binary model of gender does not represent the many ways in which gender may develop.[12]

In societies where the gender divide is not as marked, as we have discussed earlier in the book, transgender people suffer less.[13] Trans often report that a significant portion of their suffering relates to the disillusion of expectations that the significant others, initially often their parents, construct around their gender.

Gender dysphoria is in an important way a function of societal inability to contemplate alternative representations of one's identity:[14] it is thus *on a par* with other types of body dissatisfaction caused by suspect norms of social acceptability. These norms, in the some cases, are clearly morally discriminatory and racist. In the case of gender, they are not only morally dubious (they in fact condemn those with atypical gender identification to the corner of 'deviance'); they are also conceptually mistaken, as we are now going to see.

S1.3   Gender as a Social Construct

The idea that there are only two genders, fixed and stable across one's life, is a mistake: the binomial distinction of gender does not capture the diversity in which gender may develop; it also assumes that normality requires sex and gender to be congruent, and thus conjectures that biological sex is a clear datum, observable by means of empirical inspection. Under this perspective, an XX individual with primary and secondary sex characteristics congruent with genetic and chromosomal heritage (a biological female) who does not identify with the biological sex, suffers gender dysphoria. However, the biological facts are not straightforward, as we saw in Chapter 2. If biological sex was truly the standard test to assess normality, then those with DSDs should always be confused about their gender, and this is not the case. Many intersex individuals have unequivocal gender identification. Many of those with atypical gender, reversibly, often have no identifiable DSD.

Gender is, to a large extent at least, a social construct. Gender is in an important way construed around the cues (positive and negative reinforcements) provided by the significant others at a developmental stage (see Chapter 2). This has important ethical implications for medical practice.

S1.4   Ethical Implications for Medicine

If the primary cause of people's suffering is the set of unrealistic stereotypes around sex and gender, it follows that medicine should be wary of reinforcing models of 'normality' or 'acceptability' that are responsible for tribulation. Agencies with an important social influence (such as the NHS) have a responsibility not to reinforce potentially dangerous prototypes. The case of the media and anorexia nervosa is a glaring illustration of this liability: the

(continued)

SCENARIO 1 (continued)

British Medical Association (BMA) has suggested that the use of very thin models may trigger anorexia in young women, and has warned the media and the fashion industry to exhibit more realistic images of the female body;[15] in some jurisdictions, emaciated models have even been banned from the cat-walks.[16] The argument is that if models of unrealistic beauty are dangerous, there is a reason not to use them. Why shouldn't the medical profession be subjected to the same norms of moral responsibility?

The effort in the direction of dignity for all, in spite of personal arbitrary differences (such as body shape, age, and gender) should be a concerted effort by all those with public influence over people's welfare. Therefore, certainly the state should not give its support to practices that are ethically dubious and that risk reinforcing discrimination against those who are different.

If suffering is caused primarily by suspect norms, then the state should not provide support to medical practices that, implicitly, contribute to crystallising those norms. Instead, the state and civil society should attempt to change suspect norms rather than people's bodies.

S1.5   A Matter of Private Transaction?

It could be objected that even if some conditions are primarily social in nature, this does not mean that medical treatment should be denied: first, it is not always clear to what extent suffering is caused by social factors; personal variables, intra-psychic factors, even unknown biological influences may also be implicated in any disease. It cannot be up to doctors to make judgments over the authenticity of one's requests.[17] Second, all our preferences or needs are somehow influenced by society and the environment, and it is customary for medicine to intervene despite this. Infertility treatments, surgery for bat ears, and breast reconstruction following cancer treatment are only a few examples of medical interventions provided largely because of social stereotypes of 'normality': they are administered purely on psychological grounds and are often publicly funded or reimbursed under insurance schemes (see Chapter 8).[18] Denying treatments for socially determined suffering would lead to a whole recasting of medicine.[19] Third, it could be objected that whereas influential agencies have a responsibility not to spread dangerous ideals of social acceptability, individuals should not be turned into martyrs of ideals:[20] if I request skin bleaching because I experience being black as disadvantageous, it is of little help to me to be denied the treatment that would improve the quality of my life, in the name of ideals of equality or nondiscrimination in which I do not recognise myself.

For these reasons, provision of these treatments is not unethical, but it must remain within the arena of private transactions between applicants and professionals. Competent adults have significant freedom to decide what they want to do with their bodies and with their private lives: over these matters

(continued)

SCENARIO 1 (continued)

they have a *prima facie* right to absolute noninterference. Decisions relating to one's body, within the limits of duty of care and professional responsibility, should be matters relating to personal freedom and should be treated as private transactions between applicants and professionals.

S1.6 "All People Are Free in Dignity and Rights"...

. . . recites the *Universal Declaration of Human Rights*.[21] Thus, people with similar problems should be treated similarly. To fund treatment for gender issues at the expense of equally valid claims is an infringement of this important principle of ethics: not only would this imply that those other claims are less worthy of attention; it would also insinuate that people with gender dysphoria are *a case apart*. Rather than protecting and defending transgender people from discrimination and stigma, a default policy that provides publicly funded treatment for transsexualism but not for other requests of body modification reinforces the label of transsexualism as an illness, a deviance.

All desires to look more 'like oneself', to feel better in one's skin, are *on a par*: they are either all paid for or none are paid for. If only some can be paid for, then they should be chosen at random, or based on income, or on some other morally neutral criteria. Distribution in these cases should not be based on a fictional 'clinical' need, as becoming feline may be as important to the Cat Woman as a breast implant to a transsexual.

Moreover, one should ask: what are 'gender' issues? The answer to this question is not straightforward and this illustrates further how it would be unethical to publicly fund sex realignment treatment but not other body modifications.

Suppose I suffer because I have an androgynous structure: my perceived gender, my sense of who I am collides with the way I look. Mine is, of course, an issue of mismatch between my external phenotypical appearance and who I feel I am. Why should I pay for hair removal and breast implants, which relieves my mismatch, whereas females who want a penis should not pay to correct their own mismatch?

S1.7 Conclusions

The classification of gender dysphoria amongst mental illnesses in the DSM was a violation of the human right to be different, as upheld by the *Universal Declaration of Human Rights*, amongst others. But also demanding that treatment should be publicly funded is a violation of the human right to be different and to be treated equally regardless of one's arbitrary differences. In fact, offering special treatment to one category of potential applicants (transgenders) over other similar applicants, equally unhappy with the way they look, violates the human right of the latter category to be treated with equal concern and respect, and continues to condemn the group of transgenders to the stigma of being a category apart.

(continued)

SCENARIO 1 (continued)

From all this, a number of consequences follows: society has a responsibility to reduce the stigma associated with one's arbitrary features (ethnic origins, age, sex, and gender). Nonetheless, the principle of autonomy over one's body cannot and should not be abridged: people should retain the freedom to modify their body, to the extent that this causes no direct harm to others or limits an equal freedom of others. Offering publicly funded treatment to the category of transgenders at the expense of other categories of people seeking body modifications limits the equal freedom of these others; it also continues to stigmatise the category of transgenders as 'special' and 'different' from all others. Therefore, treatment for gender issues should be a matter of private transaction. Within the limits imposed by the duty of care and professional obligations, doctors and patients should negotiate desired outcomes, and patients should pay for their own treatment.

SCENARIO 2

S2.1 Felines, Star Treks, and Other Varieties: Should Doctors Do This?

A woman has undertaken several surgical interventions to look like a cat. Some people apparently ask for medical help to replicate the characters of *Star Trek*.[22]

Some want to have their tongue split into two, like snakes. Should doctors do this?

In principle, in England at least, doctors have no (legal) duty to satisfy people's requests for medical treatment. They do not have a duty to file my nose or jaws, should I wish to look like Julia Roberts, and certainly they do not have an obligation to help me look more feline. At the most, within the limits imposed by their duty of care, doctors have a legal and moral *right* to provide these treatments, provided that the applicants are capable of giving valid consent and that the treatment is in their best interests.

Whereas what is in someone's best interests may be debatable, and whereas it may be asked what my best interests may ethically impose on others, certainly omissions are not morally neutral options.[23] Doctors' right not to treat is not absolute: they generally must provide cogent moral or clinical reasons to withdraw their services.[24] As we saw in Chapter 7, in England there is no duty to rescue at law, but in other countries such a duty is recognised, and even where it is not, such absence can be contested.

Professionals, including doctors, have a *duty of care* towards their patients/clients, which imposes them not to harm those under their care, even if they are consenting adults, unless the harm is inflicted to prevent even greater harm or to produce a significant benefit. Surgery, for example, causes harm to the patient, but it is justified if it minimises greater harm or leads to the acquisition of significant benefits to the patient.

(continued)

SCENARIO 2 (continued)

The notions of 'harm' and 'benefits' should not be understood narrowly as risks/benefits of the treatment only, but should include an assessment of the overall consequences of treatment *versus* failure to administer treatment upon an applicant's welfare. For example, someone with so called body dysmorphic disorder could receive amputations, even if this is clinically unnecessary, in order to prevent greater harm.[25]

If the patient, for instance, will commit suicide unless s/he receives such an intervention, the amputation is no less of a life saving intervention than an amputation for gangrene. Arguably, in these cases it would be unethical to deny such treatment, as the likely foreseeable consequences of omission are pernicious or fatal. This obligation can in these cases be subsumed under the rule of rescue. Even in countries where such obligation is not foreseen by current laws, such a rule is one of the most important principles of ethics, and should not be abridged only because existing legislation fails to recognise it.

Let's see what this all has to do with transsexualism and access to medical treatment.

S2.2 The Case of Gender Identity

Gender dysphoria is characterised by severe and persistent discomfort with the assigned gender. Where the condition is persistent, the psychosocial adjustment of the sufferer is typically very difficult. There is high suicidal ideation amongst gender minorities (including youth), especially when timely medical treatment has not been provided. Whereas doctors have no legal obligation, at least in England, to intervene at request, it can be argued that they should provide treatment for gender dysphoria when three important conditions are met: first, the person must be in distress, and his or her suffering cannot be ameliorated with psychological/social intervention (for example, with psychotherapy or family or school involvement); second, the applicant has been assessed by specialists, and it must be sufficiently clear that the person's gender identification is atypical and that the person will benefit from medical care; finally, it should be expected that not providing treatment is the most risky option: for example, it should be probable that the overall psychosocial sequelae associated with not providing treatment is pernicious and worse for the applicant than that associated with treatment. When these conditions are met, medical intervention is ethical, and it would indeed be unethical to deny it. This should stand not only for transgenderism, but also for other types of body dissatisfaction, whether 'cosmetic', 'racial', or otherwise.

It should in fact be noted that the comparison between 'racial', 'cosmetic' surgery, and medical treatment for gender dysphoria is misleading. It suggests that, if treatment for gender dysphoria *is on a par with* 'racial' or 'cosmetic' surgery, then doctors have no moral obligation to provide it, and even a contentious moral right to satisfy the applicant's requests. Instead, here it is not a matter of *first* determining whether the intervention for gender dysphoria is (or is *on a par* with) 'cosmetic' or 'racial' interventions and *then* deciding *on that*

(continued)

SCENARIO 2 (continued)

basis whether medical treatment is ethically justified or not. Doing so begs the question as to why some requests are regarded as 'clinical needs' and others are not. Also, this is not a matter of drawing lists of demands that should or should not be fulfilled, based on the way in which these demands are qualified (as 'cosmetic' or 'racial' as opposed to 'medical'). It is instead a matter of assessing, together with the applicant, the overall expected consequences of treatment *versus not providing treatment*. Where the risk–benefit ratio appears to be in favour of medical intervention, then, *prima facie*, intervention should be provided, and society and the state have a responsibility to provide public support for requested interventions. This obligation can also be subsumed under the rule of rescue.

S2.3   Gender as a Social Construct

The suffering associated with gender dysphoria is caused to a significant extent by a suspect bipolar model of gender (see Chapter 2). Gender dysphoria is somehow construed around norms of social acceptability: these are scientifically ungrounded and also unethical, to the extent that they promote the idea that gender difference is a *deviance*. It could thus be argued that treatment for gender dysphoria is *on a par* with 'cosmetic' or 'racial' surgery, and that we shouldn't change people's bodies, we should change the social norms.

This argument reminds us of the responsibility that society has to ensure equal dignity for all, regardless of gender orientation. However, this argument misses out on some important points: first, many transsexuals do not wish *to conform to social stereotypes of masculinity or femininity*: in fact, they often depart radically from those. Many explore different gender identities in different contexts (use their female identity in some settings and their male identity in others); many take hormones to become more masculine or feminine, but want to keep their genitals. Many embrace various elements of both genders, well beyond the classic gender divide. Thus there is a difference between those who seek medical intervention *to conform* to social norms of acceptability and those who seek medical intervention against social stereotypes in order to express more fully who they are. Second, society should ensure that everybody's dignity and rights are protected regardless of arbitrary features such as race, age, and gender. But from this it does not follow that gender minorities should receive no medical care (or no funded medical care). Of course, if society is wrong we should change society. However, this does not imply that we should deny medical treatment that may also be necessary in order to ensure that everybody's differences are respected and protected. If it is possible to alleviate people's suffering, then there is a *prima facie* stringent moral reason to do so.

This has important ethical implications for medical practice.

S2.4   Ethical Implications for Medicine

Doctors perhaps have a responsibility not to reinforce mistaken norms of social acceptability (as the fashion industry and the media, for example, also have).

(continued)

SCENARIO 2 (continued)

However, they have a responsibility to alleviate people's suffering and ameliorate their quality of life. A principle of minimisation of harm and a principle of beneficence are found in virtually all moral and professional codes. The fact that a condition is partly determined by social factors should not cloud our judgment in observing and assessing that condition. Infertility is in many cases socially induced. Many women, due to social variables, seek children later in life, when their fertility decreases. In those cases, infertility is clearly a function of social factors, but this does not imply that, *for that reason*, medical treatment should not be provided and funded publicly. The state also funds medical treatment for conditions on social and psychological grounds:[26] breast reconstruction after accidents or after breast cancer, surgery for bat ears, and hormonal treatment for excessive or retarded growth are all examples of interventions meant to align the person to social standards of normality.[27] These are typically funded publicly or reimbursed under many insurance schemes.

Even if suffering is to a significant extent socially determined, it does not follow that people should not receive treatment that is proven to alleviate their affliction. Only by tempering that distress and allowing people to flourish, will the medical profession promote acceptance for people's differences.

S2.5 A Matter of Private Transaction?

Even if gender dysphoria is not an illness, treatment should not be regarded as a matter of private transaction. First, not being an illness is normatively irrelevant in this sense: it is well known that some disability right activists contested that their conditions are not disabilities but different abilities.[28] Some have tried to have deaf children, contending that deafness is indeed a privileged state.[29] This shows that the notions of disability/disorder are not just a matter of empirical or scientific observation, but a matter of value, and that their nature is elusive.

Therefore, these notions cannot be and should not be the standard test to decide whether people's claims should be satisfied and how. Moreover, the argument begs the question as to why some conditions (which appear deserving of treatment) are regarded as illnesses and others are not. Second, there are many conditions that are treated medically in spite of not being 'illnesses' (see previous section). If treatment for these conditions is offered, then *prima facie* treatment for gender dysphoria should also be offered on the same grounds: if it is likely to reduce suffering or prevent greater harm, is potentially life saving, and is likely to ameliorate the sufferer's quality of life.

S2.6 "All People Are Free in Dignity and Rights". . .

. . . recites the *Universal Declaration of Human Rights*. Thus, people with similar problems should be treated similarly. To fund treatment for gender issues at the expense of equally valid claims is, it could be argued, an infringement of this important principle of ethics. However, gender dysphoria is not *on a par* with the wish to become feline or with the unease with some of our body

(continued)

SCENARIO 2 (continued)

parts. First, for many of those affected, gender dysphoria is a terrible state to be in. If not treated, the psychological and social sequelae is for them grim and hideous (see Chapter 4). One may object that the psychosocial adjustment of the Cat Woman was very poor before becoming feline. However, there is much less evidence about the psychological dynamics and outcomes for those seeking 'racial' or 'cosmetic' (or feline) surgery. An empirical assessment of various applicants to treatment for gender dysphoria and other body modifications would be necessary before one can argue that these various conditions are *on a par* and should be treated in the same way. Second, receiving medical treatment is a life-or-death matter for many transgenders. In these cases, treatment should be regarded as life saving. Of course if rhinoplasty were to save someone's life, it should equally be regarded as life saving. Third, whereas the predilection for a smaller nose or a bigger breast can be *a preference*, it is not clear that gender dysphoria is a matter of preference in the same way. The onset of transgenderism is in many cases very early and is often persistent.[30] It is thus likely that gender dysphoria has to do with early development of gender identity rather than with the susceptibility to and acquisition of social stereotypes.

Thus, gender variance is not comparable in all morally relevant senses to other types of body discomfort. The causes of this phenomenon are unknown and are probably multiple,[31] but facts such as its severity and early onset may indicate that there is something not negotiable about atypical gender identification.

S2.7   Conclusions

Because atypical gender development is not to be regarded as an illness, therefore *it should be considered on a par with other forms of body discomfort.* This argument is incomplete. The fact that several types of body discomfort are not illnesses does not mean they are all *on a par.*

Because many types of body modifications are matters of private transaction, therefore *medical treatment for gender dysphoria must also be.* This argument is also flawed. It might well be that some other types of body modifications should also be funded publicly or reimbursed under insurance schemes.

From all this, a number of consequences follow: society has a responsibility to reduce the stigma associated with one's arbitrary features (ethnic origins, age, sex, and gender). This does not mean that all claims to body modifications deserve social support. It means that treatment (whether 'cosmetic' or otherwise) should be offered and publicly funded when the conditions discussed in the preceding are met. Whether or not medical treatment should be offered and paid for depends not on the type of condition one has, but on whether the condition (whether associated with gender, ethnic belonging, or others) is severe enough to impinge significantly upon the quality of life of the sufferer, to markedly jeopardise his or her psychosocial functioning, and whether available medical treatment is likely to ameliorate his or her condition.

5 CONCLUSIONS: WHAT WE HAVE REASON TO PREFER

The Polish film director and writer Krzysztof Kieslowsky produced a film in 1982, called *Blind Chance*, from which perhaps *Sliding Doors* took inspiration. The film splits in three, rather than two, stories. At the beginning of the film, Witek, the protagonist, runs to the station to get a train to Warsaw. He crashes into an old man who is drinking a beer. In one scenario, he ignores the fact and, in a moment, he is able to jump on the last carriage of the already moving train. In the second scenario, he just apologises quickly, but nonetheless misses the train. In the third, he stops to help the old man and misses the train. His life, from now onwards, depends on whether he apologises for spilling the beer of an old man. The paths his life takes, depending on these seemingly inconsequential facts and choices (an old man is in his way and how he decides to respond to his disappointment), are drastically different.

The moral of the film is as obvious as it is somehow disquieting: accidental facts beyond our control, combined with the moral choices we and others may make, can radically change our life. This incontrovertible truth goes often unnoticed, and the film brings it to light and compels us to think about the moral responsibility we bear when the actors are us.

In this chapter, I have wanted to highlight some of the complexities relating to the treatment of gender identity issues. Both scenarios offer seemingly plausible arguments for and against providing publicly funded treatment for gender dysphoria. But what is more important is what these parallel railways may tell us: the moral choices that the actors may make over the random facts of our life (I happen to be born black or short, or I happen to develop my gender in an atypical way in Thailand, rather than Belgium rather than in Bristol, where both society and the medical profession may make a number of diverse moral choices relating to my condition) can have a number of consequences in our own lives. In this light, it becomes imperative that we, as actors, take the course of action that, with the insight of available evidence, is likely to promote the best outcome and to minimise the risk of highly negative consequences.

We have seen in detail in the course of this book the aftermath of untreated gender dysphoria. This includes psychological, physical, and social harm. For many transsexuals, receiving proper medical treatment as well as psychological support is a life-or-death matter. Whatever other considerations may need to be addressed, there is thus a *prima facie* moral reason to provide treatment. Whereas there may be a case for reconstructing healthcare funding perhaps according to personal finances (as is the case in some countries, where people may have to pay for a share of the healthcare costs according to income[32]), and whereas certainly there is a case for improving social acceptance of gender minorities, the compelling reason to offer medical intervention is that the condition, whatever its aetiology may be, is severe, and medical treatment can make the whole difference between one life that is acceptable and relatively flourishing and another life which is condemned to overarching grief.

10 Conclusions

It all depends on the individual and the circumstances. I call for general freedom of morals, and of all the things that are not detrimental to the peace, freedom, and happiness of others.

(Claude Cahun, 1925)[1]

Every society you build will have its fringes, and on the fringes of every society, heroic and restless vagabonds will wander, with their wild and virgin thoughts.

(Renzo Novatore, 1920)[2]

I have throughout the book suggested that transgenderism can be viewed, and should be viewed, not as pathology, as deviance, or mental disorder; even less, as a form of perversion and indecent attitude. It should be viewed as the refusal of a government, a rule, or set of rules, in which the individual does not recognise himself or herself.

The quotes reported here are one by Claude Cahun, a photographer who, as we have seen in Chapter 2, has devoted a part of her work to the challenge of genders. Renzo Novatore, who wrote the second quote in the preceding, was an Italian anarchic poet: he pointed at the value of the *wandering fringes* of every society. Transgenders are sometimes referred to as gender nomads, as wandering across new latitudes and liminalities of gender. Like other nomads, transsexuals or other gender non-conforming people are often not easily accepted in the societies that have clear precepts relating to one's gender and relative roles. Like the gypsies, trans also live in some sense beyond the state. The gypsies, as is well known, do not recognise themselves, by tradition, in any nation: they only belong to themselves. This fact is scarcely and badly tolerated by the nation-states in which gypsies are allowed to enter. A nation-state cannot conceptualise the existence of people who do not recognise themselves as either citizens or foreigners. Yet nomads are not outsiders, they are just beyond the borders, beyond the recognised categories, they are like the *Frusculicchi* of Carlo Levi, neither Italians nor foreigners, neither fascists nor partisans, neither citizens nor enemies. This makes it impossible to rule them, to govern them: also for this reason, they, like trans, are usually unwelcome.

Some things cannot be governed, and gender is one of them. Any attempt to govern another person's gender according to our own ideas, assumptions, and morals represents not only a form of abuse towards the individual concerned, but a way of silencing a diversity that enriches humankind. Transgenderism involves a challenge to the rules, the norms, the customs, and the government that establish, against science and morality, that people should be either women or men, and should conform in a myriad of ways to the constellation of expectations that follow an individual through life, after a sex is assigned to them at birth.

Transgenderism is not only to be respected and understood, but to be valued. If anything, transgenderism epitomises an endeavour towards an authentic life. Across the centuries philosophy has celebrated the attainment of a life that is authentic to oneself.

"Of all human sciences", wrote Jean Jacques Rousseau, "the most useful and most imperfect appears to me to be that of mankind: and I will venture to say, the single inscription on the Temple of Delphi [know thyself] contained a precept more difficult and more important than is to be found in all the huge volumes that moralists have ever written. [. . .] How shall we know the source of inequality between men, if we do not begin by knowing mankind?" [3]

Importantly, in the last lines reported, Rousseau recognised that such knowledge is essential to the respect of human beings as formally equal, and thus to the protection of all individuals against unjust discrimination.

Respect for gender differences, with all that entails, is not to be seen only as a precept subsumed under the general liberal rules of noninterference; it is not just a claim of freedom under liberal or libertarian philosophical, political, or moral principles. Transgenderism challenges the ordinary ways in which we may think about human beings. Trangenderism requires us to rethink about what sort of beings we are.

It emerged in the course of this book that in some ways it makes little sense to inquire into the causes of transgenderism. The causes of transgenderism are, so far as we can tell, the same as the causes of all gender identities: people are who they are, and they develop through extremely complex pathways that are unique to them. Paul Goodman, an anarchist intellectual, wrote that "it is by losing ourselves in inquiry, creation and craft that we become something". [4]

For all these reasons, the approach that should be taken towards gender minorities, including (and especially) children, is one of dispassionate and compassionate understanding. This does not mean we should underestimate the trauma of parents of children with a non-conforming gender. It means instead accepting that gender may develop in unpredicted ways. Gender identity cannot be challenged: it must be a personal discovery and creation. Many people do find their gender or adapt to a gender fairly peacefully; many people need more support. They must be assisted in all possible ways in order for them to express more fully who they are, and in order to prevent and put an end to the deplorable sequelae through which many trans still have to go.

What is to be won or lost here is of great importance for the individuals concerned, but also for society as a whole. It is a known fact that transgenders are exposed to high degrees of ostracism and violence. I have reported some figures earlier in the book, but it is worth to see perhaps in greater detail the extremity of what is at stake. According to a 2003 report, from the end of 2002 to the end of 2003, thirty-eight transsexuals have been reported murdered. Following is a summary of some of these stories.[5]

On 4 December 2002 Fernanda Cavarrubias was seen leaving with a man in a red truck. Her body, mutilated and cut into pieces, was found in the river in San Felipe, in Chile.

On 14 December 2002 Tamyra Michaels, from Highland Park in Michigan, was shot by a man. She was a transwoman aged twenty-one. She died in hospital on 21 December 2002.

On 8 January 2003 Timothy Broadus, also called Cinnamon, a trans sex worker aged twenty-one, died in Fort Lauderdale, Florida. Someone driving a motorbike shot Cinnamon to death.

On 21 February 2003 Nikki Nicholas, an Afro-American trans woman aged nineteen, was found dead. She used to work as a transvestite in nightclubs around Detroit.

On 28 February 2003 Danisha Victoria Principal Williams, a transsexual, was found dead in her apartment in Brandenton, Florida. Danisha's body was left in the bath.

On 6 March 2003 the body of a transwoman from Cali, Colombia, was found thrown along a motorway. She had been stabbed to death.

On 7 March 2003 the body of Ronald Andrew Brown was found in the flat of Jason Edward Piper. She was stabbed to death. She was sixteen years old.

On 22 March 2003 Merlinka, also known as Vjeran Miladinovic, was killed in Belgrade. She was the first declared transwoman in Serbia, and she had written the book *Tereza's Son* and had worked as an actress in two Serbian films.

On 25 March 2003 Jorge Rafael Cruz was killed by a gang in Guatemala City. Jorge was a transsexual aged nineteen.

On 9 May 2003 Jessica Mercado, a twenty-four-year-old trans living in New Haven, Connecticut, was found dead. Her body was hidden under a mattress. The murderers, after killing her, set fire to the flat.

On 31 May 2003 Shelby Tracy Tom, an Asian transwoman living in Vancouver, Canada, was found dead. Her body was found in a supermarket trolley behind a laundry in North Vancouver. In this case, Jatin Patel was charged with murder.

On 22 July 2003 Nireah Johnson and Brandie Coleman were both shot in the head while sitting in a small van belonging to Brandie's mother. Nireah and Brandie lived in Indianapolis. Nireah was a transwoman. Brandie was mother to a two-month-old baby. The murderer, perhaps a man called Paul Anthony Moore, set fire to the vehicle. They were seventeen and eighteen years old.

On 7 October 2003 Adrian Torres de Assuncao died in hospital in Brescia, Italy. Adrian was a Brazilian trans aged twenty-four. A client hit Adrian in the face with a hammer. According to the report, she decided not to go to hospital because she feared that she would be sent back to Brazil, being a clandestine immigrant. When she agreed to go to hospital, it was too late.

On 16 December 2003 Georgina Matehaere, who lived in Auckland, New Zealand, was hit in the face five times with a baseball bat by Joe Tua Coleman. She died six days after.

There are many more reported cases. Many of these stories, as it will be noted, concern young people, adolescents, or very young adults. These stories call for a reflection upon the responsibilities that society as a whole has in reducing the risks for gender minorities. As explained early in the book, timely healthcare intervention is one of the ways in which such risks can be minimised. Harm reduction must be a legitimate goal of healthcare practice, together with social, political, and legal interventions. Transgenders, especially young transgenders, need to have healthcare services promptly available which assist them in the formation of their gender identity, with medication where appropriate, and prevent them from getting entangled in street life. This book has focused on the clinical encounter between trans and doctors, but as we have seen, medical intervention must be accompanied by a reform in the way people think about gender, and in the way the state, with its various agencies, accommodates gender minorities.

The World Professional Association for Transgender Health (WPATH), as we have seen in Chapter 5, also recognises harm reduction as one of the legitimate goals of the therapeutic intervention with trans. But how 'harm' should be understood can be debatable. In this book I have suggested that doctors should not think of 'harm' simply as the possible negative side effects of certain treatments: they should think of 'harm' more broadly: evaluation of harm should include an assessment of the suffering that each individual is likely to experience if s/he is not treated. The philosophers Smart and Williams pointed out that "in most cases we can do most for our fellow men by trying to remove their miseries".[6] This book has attempted to suggest reasoned ways through which each individual and all of us collectively can move towards the realisation of this legitimate ambition.

Notes

NOTES TO THE FOREWORD

1. William Shakespeare, *Twelfth Night*, in *The Arden Shakespeare*, Richard Proudfoot, Ann Thompson, and David Scott Kasten (eds.) Walton-on-Thames, Thomas Nelson and Sons, 1998, 2.4, lines 38 and 39.

NOTES TO THE PREFACE

1. Fabrizio De André, 'Marinella', in *Tutti Morimmo a Stento*, Bluebell Records, Milan, 1968.
2. Christine Korsgaard, 'Capability and Well Being', in Martha Nussbaum and Amartya Sen (eds.), *The Quality of Life*, Oxford, Oxford University Press, 1999, p. 59.

NOTES TO THE INTRODUCTION

1. Peter Dale (ed.), *Poems of François Villon, the Legacy, the Testament and Other Poems*, trans. and intro. Peter Dale, London, Anvil Press, 2001, p. 11.
2. I use the term *dis-ease* with a dash to detach the condition from pathologies, considering that the word *disease* is often used as a synonym of disorder or illness. I instead want to emphasise the lack of ease (hence dis-ease) generally associated with the condition.
3. Readapted from the poem "To Signs" (1913) by Vladimir Majakovskij. An English version of the poem, with a commentary, can be found in J. R. Stapanian, 'V. Majakovskij's "To Signs" (Vyveskam)—a Cubist "Signboard" in Verse', *Slavic and East European Journal*, 26, 2, 1982, pp. 174–86.
4. Francesco Guccini, 'Autogrill', in Francesco Guccini, *Guccini*, EMI, 1983.
5. Fabrizio De André, 'Via del Campo', in *Volume I*, Bluebell Records, Milano, 1967.

NOTES TO CHAPTER 1

1. Hans Christian Andersen, *The Little Mermaid*, 1836. Online at http://hca.gilead.org.il/li_merma.html. The passage cited in this chapter is readapted from the translation of this site. Last accessed 19 December 2011.

2. GLSEN, Education Department Resource, "Celebrating Lesbian Gay Bisexual Transgender (LGBT) History Month, 2001". Online at http://www.glsen.org/binary-data/GLSEN_ATTACHMENTS/file/181–1.pdf. Last accessed 1 July 2011. See also Jackie Wullschläger, *Hans Christian Andersen: The Life of a Storyteller*, New York, Knopf, 2001.
3. L. Weitzman et al., 'Sexual Socialization in Picture Books for Preschool Children', *American Journal of Sociology*, 77, 1972, pp. 1125–50.
4. Another interesting study on fairy tales is that by Madonna Kolbenschlag, *Kiss Sleeping Beauty Good-Bye: Breaking the Spell of Feminine Myths and Models*, Garden City, Doubleday, 1979.
5. B. Davies, *Frogs and Snails and Feminist Tales*, Sydney, Allen and Unwin, 1991; A. Pisetta, *Genere e socializzazione scolastica. Una ricerca sulla rappresentazione dei modelli sessuali nei libri di testo per le elementary*, Tesi di Laurea, Università degli Studi di Trento, 2004. Online at http://www.tesionline.it/consult/indice.jsp?idt=11470. Last accessed 9 May 2012. Cited in Elisabetta Ruspini, *Le Identità di Genere*, Milan, Carocci, 2009, p. 79.
6. Ruspini, *Le Identità di Genere*, p. 83.
7. Ibid., p. 84.
8. Ibid.
9. Janice G. Raymond, *The Transsexual Empire. The Making of the She-Male*, London, Teachers College Press, 1994, p. 79.
10. Leslies Feinberg, *Trans Gender Warriors, Making History from Joan of Arc to Dennis Rodman*, Boston, Beacon Press, 1996, p. x.
11. Raymond, *Transsexual Empire*, p. 12.
12. This point is made, for example, by Besnier, who, however, also argues that this assumption is mistaken: "as sociolinguists have argued, grammatical gender is largely unrelated to social gender, and the presence or absence of the former says nothing about the nature of the latter". See Niko Besnier, 'Polynesian Gender Liminality through Time and Space, in Gilbert Herdt (ed.), *Third Sex Third Gender, beyond Sexual Dimorphism in Culture and History*, New York, Zone Books, 1996, pp. 285–328, p. 305.
13. Richard Ekins and Dave King, 'Pioneers of Transgendering: The Popular Sexology of David O. Cauldwell', *International Journal of Transgenderism*, Special Issue on David O. Cauldwell (1897–1959), 5, 2, April–June 2001. Online at http://www.wpath.org/journal/www.iiav.nl/ezines/web/IJT/97–03/numbers/symposion/cauldwell_01.htm. Last accessed 1 July 2011.
14. Frank Lewins, *Transsexualism in Society. A Sociology of Male-to-Female Transsexuals*, Melbourne, MacMillan, 1995, p. 21. The study cited is William A. W. Walters and Michael W. Ross (eds.), *Transsexualism and Sex Reassignment*, Melbourne, Oxford University Press, 1986.
15. For Benjamin, transsexualism (and transvestism) was a symptom of an underlying psychopathology of sex or gender role disorientation. See Anne Bolin, "Transcending and Transgendering: Male-to-Female Transsexuals, Dichotomy and Diversity", in Gilbert Herdt (ed.), *Third Sex Third Gender, beyond Sexual Dimorphism in Culture and History*, New York, Zone Books, 1996, pp. 447–486, p. 455.
16. Robert Mills, "Queer is Here? Lesbian, Gay, Bisexual and Transgender Histories and Public Culture", *History Workshop Journal*, 62, 1, 2006, pp. 253–63.
17. Jan Morris, *Conundrum*, London, Faber and Faber, 1974, pp. 35–38.
18. D. Di Ceglie, "Management and Therapeutic Aims in Working with Children and Adolescents with Gender Identity Disorders, and Their Families", in D. Di Ceglie and D. Freedman (eds.), *A Stranger in My Own Body—Atypical*

Gender Identity Development and Mental Health, London, Karnac Books, 1998, chap. 12, pp. 185–97, p. 185.

19. A picture is available online at http://www.lib-art.com/imgpainting/0/1/19310–night-michelangelo-buonarroti.jpg. Last accessed 30 May 2011.
20. Morris, *Conundrum*, p. 40.
21. See Gert Hekma, 'A Female Soul in a Male Body: Sexual Inversion as Gender Inversion in Nineteenth-Century Sexology', in Gilbert Herdt (ed.), *Third Sex Third Gender, beyond Sexual Dimorphism in Culture and History*, New York, Zone Books, 1996, pp. 213–39.
22. An account of some of those may be found in Randolph Trumbach, "London's Sapphists: From Three Sexes to Four Genders in the Making of Modern Culture", in Gilbert Herdt (ed.), *Third Sex Third Gender, beyond Sexual Dimorphism in Culture and History*, New York, Zone Books, 1996, pp. 111–36.
23. Brian Booth and Thomas Lauderdale, 'Alberta Lucille Hart/Dr. Alan L. Hart: An Oregon "Pioneer"', Oregon Cultural Heritage Commission, 2000. Online at www.ochcom.org/hart. Last accessed 4 August 2011.
24. See http://en.wikipedia.org/wiki/Lili_Elbe. Last accessed 4 August 2011.
25. Roberta Cowell, *Roberta Cowell's Story*, London, Heinemann, 1954.
26. *Corbett v. Corbett* [1971] P 83 (HL).
27. See http://www.legislation.gov.uk/ukpga/2004/7/contents. Last accessed 20 September 2011.
28. Raymond, *Transsexual Empire*, p. xix.
29. Eric Meininger and Gary Ramafedi, 'Gay, Lesbian, Bisexual and Transgender Adolescents', in Lawrence S. Neinstein (ed.), *Adolescent Health Care: A Practical Guide*, Minneapolis, Lippincott Williams and Wilkins, 2008, chap. 40.
30. See, for example, Bernard Reed, Stephene Rhodes, Pietà Schofield, and Kevan Wylie, *Gender Variance in the UK: Prevalence, Incidence, Growth and Geographic Distribution*, London, Gender Identity Research and Education Society, 2009, in particular pp. 31ff.
31. See http://www.traditionalvalues.org/pdf_files/TVCSpecialRptTransgenders1234.PDF. Last accessed 13 May 2011.
32. D. Di Ceglie, 'Reflections on the Nature of the "Atypical Gender Identity Organization"', in D. Di Ceglie and D. Freedman (eds.), *A Stranger in My Own Body—Atypical Gender Identity Development and Mental Health*, London, Karnac Books, 1998, chap. 2, pp. 9–25.
33. Bolin, 'Transcending and Transgendering', pp. 447–486, p. 447.
34. I refer to children and adolescents without defining a clear cut age at which a child becomes an adolescent.

NOTES TO CHAPTER 2

1. Emile Durkheim, *The Elementary Forms of the Religious Life (1912)*, Oxford, Oxford University Press, 2001, p. 13.
2. Aristotle, *Topics* 102 *a* 31. The *Topics* is the name given by Aristotle to his works on logic, which include the *Categories* cited in the following. One edition is translated by W. A. Pickard-Cambridge, published by eBooks@ Adelaide and available online at http://ebooks.adelaide.edu.au/a/aristotle/a8t/. Last accessed 20 December 2011.
3. There are many editions of the *Sophist*. One is *Plato's Sophist: A Translation with a Detailed Account of Its Theses and Arguments*, trans. James Duerlinger, New York, Lang, 2005.

4. Again, there are many editions of the *Categories*. One is *Aristotle's Categories, and De interpretazione*, trans. with notes by J. L. Ackrill, Oxford, Clarendon Press, 1990.
5. John Archer and Barbara Lloyd, *Sex and Gender*, Cambridge, Cambridge University Press, 2002, p. 17; see also M. Boylan, 'The Galenic and Hippocratic Challenges to Aristotle's Conception Theories', *Journal of the History of Biology*, 17, 1984, pp. 83–112.
6. Gayle Rubin, 'The Traffic in Women. Notes on the Political Economy of Sex', in R. Reiter (ed.), *Towards an Anthropology of Women*, New York, Monthly Review Press, 1975, pp. 157–210.
7. Archer and Lloyd, *Sex and Gender*, p. 17.
8. Clearly sociology and feminist/gender studies encompass a great variety of approaches and expertise. I do not pretend to offer here an accurate account of what sociologists, feminists, and specialists in gender studies have explained about gender. I only wish to portray in broad lines the contribution of these humanistic disciplines to the understanding of gender and gender identity. Later in the chapter we will see how differently gender identity is understood in 'scientific' disciplines, such as endocrinology and clinical psychology.
9. Elisabetta Ruspini, *Le Identità di Genere*, Milan, Carocci, 2009, p. 18.
10. Rubin, 'Traffic in Women'.
11. Frank Lewins, *Transsexualism in Society. A Sociology of Male-to-Female Transsexuals*, Melbourne, MacMillan Education, 1995, pp. 33–34.
12. David E. Grimm, 'Toward a Theory of Gender: Transsexualism, Gender, Sexuality and Relationships', *American Behavioral Scientist*, 31, 1, 1987, pp. 66–85, p. 81.
13. Joan W. Scott, "Gender: A Useful Category of Historical Analysis", *American Historical Review*, 91, 5, 1986, pp. 1053–75. Online at http://www.cedis.uni-koeln.de/content/e310/e625/Text1frWorkshopzurHermeneutischenDialoganalyse_gender_ger.pdf. Last accessed 31 July 2011.
14. Ruspini, *Le Identità di Genere*, p. 11.
15. R. Gross, *Psychology*, 6th edition, London, Hodder Education, 2010. See also http://psychology.jrank.org/pages/1735/sexual-development.html. Last accessed 30 May 2011.
16. Randy J. Nelson, *An Introduction to Behavioral Endocrinology*, 3rd ed., Sunderland, MA, Sinauer Associates, 2005, p. 109.
17. Gross, *Psychology*, p. 563.
18. Rosario A. Vernon, "Intersex and the Molecular Deconstruction of Sex", *Journal of Lesbian and Gay Studies*, 15, 2009, pp. 267–83, p. 269. I owe this observation to Melanie Newbould.
19. Melanie Newbould, unpublished.
20. I wish to thank Melanie Newbould for the references and the considerations briefly summarised in these lines.
21. Kiira Triea, *Hasting Center Report, Bioethics Forum*, 2010. Online at http://www.thehastingscenter.org/Bioethicsforum/Post.aspx?id=4426. Last accessed 30 May 2011.
22. Nelson, *Introduction*, see in particular chaps. 3 and 4.
23. Gross, *Psychology*, p.566.
24. Avicenna, *De hermaphrodito*, in the *Canon Medicinae*, Liber III, Fen XX, Tractatus I, chap. 43, Venetiis: apud Iuntas, 1608.
25. I wish to thank Monica Santoro and Dino Topi for helping with the translation from the original.
26. B. Mendonca, S. Domenice, I. J. P. Arnhold, and E. M. F. Costa, '46, XY Disorders of Sex Development—DSD', *Clinical Endocrinology*, 70, 2, 2009, pp. 173–87.

27. Milton Diamond and Linda Ann Watson, 'Androgen Insensitivity Syndrome and Klinefelter's Syndrome: Sex and Gender Considerations', *Child and Adolescent Psychiatric Clinics, of North America*, 13, 2004, pp. 623–40.
28. Anne Fausto-Sterling, 'The Five Sexes: Why Male and Female Are Not Enough', *The Sciences*, March/April 1993, pp. 20–21. As cited in Leslies Feinberg, *Trans Gender Warriors, Making History from Joan of Arc to Dennis Rodman*, Boston, Beacon Press, 1996, p. 101.
29. Intersex Society of North America, *What Is Intersexy?*, San Francisco, Intersex Society of North America. Online at http://www.isna.org/faq/what_is_ intersex Last accessed 9 May 2012.
30. Gilbert Herdt, 'Introduction: Third Sexes and Third Genders', in Gilbert Herdt (ed.), *Third Sex Third Gender, beyond Sexual Dimorphism in Culture and History*, New York, Zone Books, 1996, p. 25.
31. Ibid., p. 34.
32. Ibid., p. 56.
33. Lewins, *Transsexualism in Society*, in particular pp. 35–37. The schema that follows is readapted from the one found in Lewins's book at p. 36.
34. Herdt, 'Introduction', p. 21.
35. Readapted from Melanie Blackless, Anthony Charuvastra, Amanda Derryck, Anne Fausto-Sterling, Karl Lauzanne, and Ellen Lee, 'How Sexually Dimorphic Are We? Review and Synthesis', *American Journal of Human Biology*, 12, 2000, pp. 151–66.
36. R. W. Connell, *Masculinities*, 2nd ed., Cambridge, Polity Press, 2005.
37. P. J. Cabanis, *Rapports du physique et du moral de l'homme*, 1824. The original version is available online in French at http://www.archive.org/ stream/rapportsduphysi01caba#page/n5/mode/2up. Last accessed 31 July 2011. My translation.
38. In F. M. Voltaire, *Dialogues et Anecdotes philosophiques*, Paris, Garnier, 1955, pp. 213–16.
39. J. F. Hegel, *Filosofia del diritto*, Italian translation by F. Messineo, Laterza, Bari, 1954, para. 166, p. 153. My translation from the Italian.
40. A. Comte, *Discorso preliminare sull'insieme del positivismo*, in *Opuscopi di Filosofia Sociale*, Italian translation by A. Negri, Firenze, Sansoni, 1969, p. 425ff. See in particular p. 646. My translation from the Italian.
41. S. de Beauvoir, *Le Deixoème Sex*, Paris, Gallimard, 1949.
42. John Stuart Mill, *The Subjection of Women*, 1869. Online at http://www. constitution.org/jsm/women.htm. Last accessed 31 July 2011.
43. Ibid.
44. K. Marx and F. Engels, *La Sacra Famiglia*, Italian translation by De Caria, Rome, Rinascita, 1954, p. 208. My translation from the Italian.
45. C. Fourier, *Le nouveau monde industriel et sociétaire*, Paris, Andropos, 1967–1968, vol. VI, p. 201.
46. Frederick Engels, *The Origin of the Family, Private Property and the State*, 1884, trans. Ernest Untermann, Honolulu, University Press of the Pacific, 2001, chap. 2.
47. Lewis Henry Morgan, *Ancient Society*, 1877, London, New Brunswick, 2000.
48. Frederick Engels, *The Origin of the Family, Private Property and the State*, (1884) translated by Ernest Untermann, University Press of the Pacific, Honolulu, 2001, chap. 2. An online version can be found at http://www.marxists. org/archive/marx/works/1884/origin-family/ch02c.htm Last accessed 9 May 2102
49. V. I. Lenin, *Capitalism and Female Labour*, in *Lenin Collected Works*, 1913, Moscow, Progress Publishers, 1971, vol. 36, pp. 230–31. Translation by Andrew Rothstein.

50. As stressed in this chapter there is within feminism a movement according to which it is true that women are biologically different from men and biologically 'wired' to mothering, nurturing, and care. However, this movement insists on a renewed evaluation of these roles and differences. See Ruspini, *Le Identità di Genere*, pp. 58ff.
51. Or compels me; I am not in fact arguing that the process comes without its disadvantages.
52. Kenneth J. Zucker, 'Biological Influences on Psychosexual Differentiation', in Rhoda K. Unger (ed.), *Psychology of Women and Gender*, New York, John Wiley and Sons, 2001, p. 102.
53. Eric Meininger and Gary Ramafedi, 'Gay, Lesbian, Bisexual and Transgender Adolescents', in Lawrence S. Neinstein (ed.), *Adolescent Health Care: A Practical Guide*, Minneapolis, Lippincott Williams and Wilkins, 2008, chap. 40.
54. John Money and Anke A. Ehrhardt, *Man & Woman, Boy & Girl*, Baltimore, Johns Hopkins University Press, 1972, p. 4.
55. It could be argued that the differentiation of these two characterisations of gender identity is not as stark as this. It is in fact possible that 'a body' symbolises 'a set of roles and rules'. It is thus possible that incongruence with one's external phenotype is somehow expressive of a more general sense of incongruence with all that 'having that body' entails. The same reasoning can apply to cases of ambivalent gender identification, where people feel they have both masculine and feminine sides to their selves.
56. D. Di Ceglie and D. Freedman (eds.), *A Stranger in My Own Body—Atypical Gender Identity Development and Mental Health*, London, Karnac Books, 1998.
57. Janice G. Raymond, *The Transsexual Empire. The Making of the She-Male*, London, Teachers College Press, 1994.
58. Patricia Allmer considers these artists 'surrealist', in the sense of belonging to the intellectual movement initiated by André Bréton and called 'surrealism'. I will not discuss here whether she is right or wrong to classify these artists as such. Frida Khalo, for example, included in the collection, apparently did not like surrealism and did not consider herself a surrealist. However, I suspect Allmer is using the term *surrealism* broadly, to denote a movement oblivious to boundaries.
59. Kimberley Marwood, 'Angels of Anarchy: Women, Artists and Surrealism', *Papers of Surrealism*, 8, 2010, p. 1.
60. Patricia Allmer, 'Of Fallen Angels and Angels of Anarchy', in Patricia Allmer (ed.), *Angels of Anarchy: Women Artists and Surrealism*, London, Prestel, 2009, p. 12.
61. Ibid.; see Marwood, 'Angels of Anarchy', p. 1.
62. Donna Haraway, 'A Cyborg Manifesto: Science, Technology and Socialist-Feminism in the Late Twentieth Century', in Donna Haraway (ed.), *Simians, Cyborgs and Women: The Reinvention of Nature*, London, Free Association Books, 1991, p. 181.
63. Claire Colebrook, 'Introduction', in Ian Buchanan and Claire Colebrook (eds.), *Deleuze and Feminist Theory*, Edinburgh, Edinburgh University Press, 2000, p. 4.
64. Allmer, 'Of Fallen Angels', p. 14.
65. Mary Ann Caws, 'These Photographing Women: The Scandal of Genius', in Patricia Allmer (ed.), *Angels of Anarchy: Women Artists and Surrealism*, London, Prestel, 2009, p. 30.
66. A photo of the artwork is available online at http://www.tate.org.uk/modern/exhibitions/surrealism/room3.htm. Last accessed 19 September 2011.

67. A photograph of the artwork is available online at www.leemiller.co.uk. Last accessed 19 September 2011.
68. Allmer, 'Of Fallen Angels', p. 20. A photograph of the artwork is available online at http://www.tate.org.uk/servlet/ViewWork?cgroupid=999999961& workid=2531. Last accessed 19 September 2011.
69. Allmer, 'Of Fallen Angels', p. 21.
70. An image is online at http://www.tate.org.uk/servlet/ViewWork?cgroupid=9 99999961&workid=25977. Last accessed 31 August 2011.
71. An English translation is online at http://www.poetryfoundation.org/ poem/179212. Last accessed 31 August 2011.
72. Katharine Conley, 'Safe as Houses: Anamorphic Bodies in Ordinary Spaces: Miller, Varo, Tanning, Woodman', in Patricia Allmer (ed.), *Angels of Anarchy: Women Artists and Surrealism*, London, Prestel, 2009, pp. 46–53.
73. A photograph of *House 3* is available online at http://photoworld.splinder. com/tag/autori+francesca+woodman. Last accessed 20 September 2011.
74. An image of the artwork is available online at http://www.artkernel. com/?p=3103. Last accessed 20 September 2011.
75. Quote reported at the *Claude Cahun Exhibition* in Barcelona, December 2011.

NOTES TO CHAPTER 3

1. Fabrizio De André and Ivano Fossati, 'Princesa', in *Anime Salve*, BMG Ricordi, 1996. My translation from the Italian.
2. Her biography was published in 1994. See Maurizio Jannelli, *Fernanda Farías de Albuquerque Princesa*, Milan, Editrice Sensibili alle Foglie, 1994.
3. See Simona Giordano, *Understanding Eating Disorders*, Oxford, Oxford University Press, 2005, chap. 1.
4. Richard Gross, *Psychology*, London, Hodder Education, 6th ed., 2010, pp. 571–73.
5. D. Khun, S. C. Nash, and L. Brucken, 'Sex Role Concepts of Two- and Three-Year-Olds', *Child Development*, 49, 2, 1978, pp. 445–51.
6. Richard Gross, *Psychology*, p. 573.
7. A comprehensive analysis of the strengths and weaknesses of each of these theories is provided by Gross, *Psychology*, chap. 36.
8. 'Social constructionism' is a broad philosophical term used to cover various discourses: it refers to the relationship between signifier and signified in language and to the epistemological validity of the notion of mental illness, and social constructionism as it applies to gender studies is only one portion of a broader metaphysical theory. One of the core ideas of at least several types of social constructionist theories is that some objects are products of social practices, and that these social practices are at times unacknowledged. Thus, for example, things such as race, gender, and mental illness are not biological events to which the referent gives a name, but the result of culture or social practices. Thus the metaphysical explanation for the existence of a different kind is that this is a social construct and not a biological datum. In the case of gender identity, in simple terms, constructionism assumes that gender identity is moulded by cultural models, and therefore it is relative to culture, place, historical time, and other variables. A clear and comprehensive account of social constructionism can be found open access at http://plato.stanford.edu/ entries/social-construction-naturalistic/. Last accessed 30 June 2011. References can also be found here.

9. 'Deconstructionism' should be differentiated from social constructionism. Deconstructionism is a theory most often associated with the philosopher Jacques Derrida. Deconstructionism is a critical approach to texts (words, symbols, and works of arts, for example). At a very basic level, deconstructionism points at the fact that between the signifier and the text there is an incommensurable gap. Texts, words, for example, are not static, and meanings refer to the subjective and relative interpretation that each subject gives to the texts. Given that agents/signifiers are also different, deconstructionism operates an irreducible recognition of otherness. Feminist analyses of the sexed body and of gender have stressed how the feminine body and gender are socially constructed. From this point of view, whereas the philosophical background of 'deconstructionism' should be differentiated from 'social constructionism', in gender studies and feminism they can be used as synonymous. To read more on feminists' critiques of Michael Foucault see http:// plato.stanford.edu/entries/femapproach-continental/. Last accessed 30 June 2011. This provides an easy, accessible, and comprehensive account of how feminism has somehow found its roots in the deconstructionism theory and, in particular, in Foucault's work on sex.

10. An illustrative example of feminist critique of gender differences is provided by Rachel T. Hare-Mustin and Jeanne Marecek (eds.), *Making a Difference: Psychology and the Construction of Gender*, New Haven, Yale University Press, 1990. This book explores in particular post-modernism and constructionism. See also Elisabetta Ruspini, *Le Identità di Genere*, Milan, Carocci, 2009, pp. 58ff.

11. A. Comte, "Influenza femminile del positivismo", *Sull'insieme del Positivismo*, Parte quarta, p. 624, at 228. My translation.

12. Ibid., p. 640, at 244. My translation.

13. John Bowlby, *Attachment and Loss*, vol. 1, *Attachment*, Harmondsworth, Penguin, 1969.

14. Simon Baron-Cohen, *The Essential Difference: Men, Women and the Extreme Male Brain*, London, Penguin/Basic Books, 2003, p. 1.

15. L. Fenson, V. A. Marchman, D. J. Thal, P. S. Dale, J. S. Reznick, and E. Bates, *MacArthur-Bates Communicative Development Inventories: User's Guide and Technical Manual*, 2nd ed., Baltimore, Paul H. Brookes Publishing, 2007; E. E. Maccoby and C. N. Jacklin, *The Psychology of Sex Difference*, Stanford, CA, Stanford University Press, 1974; D. N. Ruble and C. L. Martin, 'Gender Development', in W. Damon and N. Eisenberg (eds.), *Handbook of Child Psychology*, vol. 3, New York, Wiley, 1998; H. R. Schaffer, *Introducing Child Psychology*, Oxford, Blackwell, 2004.

16. Richard Green, 'Gender Identity Disorder in Children and Adolescents', in Michael G. Gelder, Nancy C. Andreasen, Juan J. Lopex-Ibor, and John R. Geddes (eds.), *New Oxford Textbook of Psychiatry*, 2nd ed., Oxford, Oxford University Press, 2009, chap. 9.

17. See ibid. for a more detailed review of these studies.

18. Randy J. Nelson, *An Introduction to Behavioral Endocrinology*, 3rd ed., Sunderland, MA, Sinauer Associates, 2005, chap. 4, in particular pp. 230–32.

19. Kenneth J. Zucker, 'Biological Influences on Psychosexual Differentiation', in Rhoda K. Unger (ed.), *Psychology of Women and Gender*, New York, John Wiley and Sons, 2001, p. 110.

20. Carol Gilligan, *In a Different Voice*, 6th ed., Cambridge, MA, Harvard University Press, 1993.

21. Joan W. Scott, 'Gender: A Useful Category of Historical Analysis', *American Historical Review*, 91, 5, 1986, pp. 1053–75. Available online at http://

www.cedis.uni-koeln.de/content/e310/e625/Text1frWorkshopzurHerme-
neutischenDialoganalyse_gender_ger.pdf. Last accessed 30 June 2011.
22. Luce Irigaray, *Speculum of the Other Woman*, trans. Gillian C. Gill, Ithaca,
NY, Cornell University Press, 1985; Luce Irigaray, *The Sex which Is Not
One*, trans. Catherine Porter, Ithaca, NY, Cornell University Press, 1985.
23. Judith Butler, *Gender Trouble: Feminism and the Subversion of Identity*,
New York, Routledge, 1989; Judith Butler, *Bodies that Matter: On the Dis-
cursive Limits of "Sex"*, New York, Routledge, 1993; Judith Butler, *The
Psychic Life of Power: Theories of Subjection*, Stanford, CA, Stanford University Press, 1997; Judith Butler, 'A "Bad Writer" Bites Back', *New York
Times*, 20 March 1999, p. 15.
24. Leslie Feinberg, *Trans Gender Warriors, Making History from Joan of Arc
to Dennis Rodman*, Boston, Beacon Press, 1996, p. 125.
25. Anne Fausto-Sterling, 'The Five Sexes: Why Male and Female Are Not
Enough', *The Sciences*, March/April 1993, pp. 23–24, as cited in Feinberg,
Trans Gender Warriors, p. 103.
26. Margaret Mead, *Male and Female*, New York, Harper Perennial, 2001; see
also Anne Fausto- Sterling, *Myths of Gender: Biological Theories about
Men and Women*, New York, Basic Books, 1985. Here the author analyses
several biological theories of gender and criticises them, showing their flaws.
She concludes that the causes for gender differences are to be found in psychology and in sociology, not in biology.
27. See, for example, Ruspini, *Le Identità di Genere*, p. 59.
28. M. Foucault, *Storia della sessualità*, vol. I, *La volontà di sapere*, 1976,
Milan, Feltrinelli, 1999,; see also J. Derrida, *Of Grammatology*, 1967, Baltimore, Johns Hopkins University Press, 1997; J. Derrida, *Spurs: Nietzsche's
Styles*, 1978, London, University of Chicago Press, 1981.
29. Judith Lorber, *Paradoxes of Gender*, London, Yale University Press, 1994.
30. See, for example, Ruspini, *Le Identità di Genere*, p. 73.
31. Green, 'Gender Identity Disorder', chap. 9. Green also produced interesting
observations of the association between homosexuality and the relationship
between fathers and sons. See Richard Green, *The 'Sissy Boy Syndrome' and
the Development of Homosexuality*, New Haven, Yale University Press, 1987.
32. A comprehensive account of socialisation is found in John Archer and Barbara Lloyd, *Sex and Gender*, Cambridge, Cambridge University Press, 2002,
pp. 60–71. Archer and Lloyd also offer an interesting critical account of
Kohlberg's theory of gender identity development and gender constancy at
pp. 66–69.
33. J. A. Will, P. Self, and N. Datan, 'Maternal Behavior and Perceived Sex of
Infant', *American Journal of Orthopsychiatry*, 46, 1976, pp. 135–39.
34. For a commentary, see Anthony Giddens and Simon Griffiths, *Sociology*, 5th
ed., Cambridge, Polity Press, 2006, p. 170. Giddens here reports and comments upon Will et al.'s study. See Will, Self, and Datan, 'Maternal Behavior', pp. 135–39.
35. Lorber, *Paradoxes of Gender*.
36. Albert Bandura, 'Influence of Model's Reinforcement Contingencies on the
Acquisition of Imitative Responses', *Journal of Personality and Social Psychology*, 1, 1965, pp. 589–95.
37. Holly Devor, *Gender Blending: Confronting the Limits of Duality*, Bloom-
ington, Indiana University Press, 1989. In a study of masculine stereotypes,
Miedzian argues that traits such as being tough, dominant, macho, and cal-
lous towards women, for example, are not natural for boys, but are socially
instigated. See Myriam Miedzian, *Boys Will Be Boys: Breaking the Link
between Masculinity and Violence*, New York, Doubleday, 1991.

38. Kay Bussey and Albert Bandura, 'Self-Regulatory Mechanisms Governing Gender Development', *Child Development*, 63, 1992, pp. 1236–50.
39. Barbara Lloyd and Gerald Duveen, 'A Semiotic Analysis of the Development of Social Representations of Gender', in Gerald Duveen and Barbara Lloyd (eds.), *Social Representations and the Development of Knowledge*, Cambridge, Cambridge University Press, 1990, chap. 3, pp. 27–46.
40. It is worth mentioning here two important books by Money. One is John Money, *Gendermaps: Social Constructionism, Feminism, and Sexosophical History*, New York, Continuum, 1995. Here Money discusses sex roles as those behaviours that are assigned by each culture on the basis of biological sex. Money rearticulates here some of his previous arguments in a way that is more accessible to the wider audience. See also John Money and Anke A. Ehrhardt, *Man & Woman, Boy & Girl*, Baltimore, Johns Hopkins University Press, 1972. Here we have a strong argument that the differences between men and women are social constructs and are not based on biology; see also John Money (ed.), *Venuses Penises: Sexology, Sexosophy, and Exigency Theory*, Buffalo, NY, Prometheus Books, 1986.
41. A more accurate analysis of John Money's theory and practice can be found in Janice G. Raymond, *The Transsexual Empire. The Making of the She-Male*, London, Teachers College Press, 1994, pp. 44–68. Here Raymond claims that Money alternatively presents gender as a biological datum or as a social construct, or as a language, that depends on some biological capacities that are 'activated' by social cues. Raymond offers a critical analysis of Money's theories.
42. Gross, *Psychology*, p. 566.
43. Zucker, 'Biological Influences', p. 105. See also Kenneth J. Zucker and Susan J. Bradley, 'Gender Identity and Psychosexual Disorders', *Focus*, 3, Fall 2005, pp. 598–617 (reprinted with permission from K. J. Zucker and S. J. Bradley, 'Gender Identity and Psychosexual Disorders', in J. M. Wiener and M. K. Dulcan [eds.], *The American Psychiatric Publishing Textbook of Child and Adolescent Psychiatry*, 3rd ed., Washington, DC, American Psychiatric Publishing, 2004, chap. 44, pp. 813–35). See also John Money and Patricia Tucker, *Sexual Signatures: On Being a Man or a Woman*, Boston, Little, Brown, 1975. In this book Money and Tucker report their clinical experience. They describe a number of cases of children with anomalies of sex development (now called DSDs), showing how these have developed satisfactory gender identification. They interpret this evidence as meaning that culture strongly shapes gender identification.
44. A more recent suggestion relating to treatment of intersex children can be found in J. K. Hewitt and G. L. Warne, 'Management of Disorders of sex Development', *Pediatric Health*, 3, 1, 2009, pp. 51–65.
45. John Colapinto, *As Nature Made Him: The Boy Who Was Raised as A Girl*, New York, HarperCollins, 2000. For a more recent dispute on medical treatment for a child with CAH, see H. F. Meyer-Bahlburg and F. L. Heino, 'Male Gender Identity in an XX Individual with Congenital Adrenal Hyperplasia', *Journal of Sexual Medicine*, 6, 1, 2009, pp. 297–98; see also Juan Carlos Jorge, Carolina Echeverri, Yailis Medina, and Pedro Acevedo, 'Male Gender Identity in an XX Individual with Congenital Adrenal Hyperplasia: A Response by the Authors', *Journal of Sexual Medicine*, 6, 1, 2009, pp. 298–99.
46. Noa Ben-Asher, 'Paradoxes of Health and Equality: When a Boy Becomes a Girl', *Yale Journal of Law & Feminism*, 16, 2004, pp. 275–312.
47. See the Intersex Society of North America at http://www.isna.org/faq/patient-centered. Last accessed 30 June 2011.

48. Melanie Newbould, *Legal and Ethical Issues Surrounding Infantile and Childhood Genital Surgery*, doctoral thesis in Bioethics and Medical Jurisprudence, University of Manchester, work in progress.
49. Kenneth J. Zucker, 'Intersexuality and Gender Identity Differentiation', *Journal of Pediatric and Adolescent Gynecology*, 15, 1, 2002, pp. 3–13. Available online at http://www.sciencedirect.com/science?_ob=ArticleURL&_udi=B6W68-459BBNY-2&_user=494590&_coverDate=02%2F28%2F2002&_rdoc=1&_fmt=high&_orig=search&_sort=d&_docanchor=&view=c&_searchStrId=1322036193&_rerunOrigin=google&_acct=C000024058&_version=1&_urlVersion=0&_userid=494590&md5=d45b4de015ea6a95569 5c5d29488a317. Last accessed 30 June 2011. See also Wilson C. J. Chung, Gert J. De Vries, and Dick F. Swaab, 'Sexual Differentiation of the Bed Nucleus of the Stria Terminalis in Humans May Extend into Adulthood', *Journal of Neuroscience*, 22, 3, 2002, pp. 1027–33; F. P. Kruijver, J. N. Zhou, C. W. Pool, M. A. Hofman, L. J. Gooren, and D. F. Swaab, 'Male-to-Female Transsexuals Have Female Neuron Numbers in a Limbic Nucleus', *Journal of Clinical Endocrinology and Metabolism*, 85, 5, 2000, pp. 2034–41; P. J. Van Kesteren, L. J. Gooren, and J. A. Megens, 'An Epidemiological and Demographic Study of Transsexuals in the Netherlands', *Archives of Sexual Behaviour*, 25, 6, 1996, pp. 589–600; J. N. Zhou, M. A. Hofman, L. J. Gooren, and D. F. Swaab, 'A Sex Difference in the Human Brain and Its Relation to Transsexuality', *Nature*, 378, 6552, 1995, pp. 68–70.
50. From Archer and Lloyd, *Sex and Gender*, pp. 75–76.
51. Gross, *Psychology*, chap. 33.
52. Kay Deaux and Abigail J. Stewart, 'Framing Gender Identities', in Rhoda K. Unger (ed.), *Handbook of the Psychology of Women and Gender*, Wiley, 2001, chap. 6, p. 85.
53. One implication of this is that, at least to some extent, sexual and gender 'deviance' (homosexuality as well as transsexuality) is generated by normative models of sexual and gender 'normalcy'. In this sense, the 'anomaly' is created by cultural and social norms and expectations.
54. They are 'legitimate' in two senses: because their existence can be explained and justified with reason, and ethically legitimate because they concern the individual only.
55. Anne Bolin, 'Transcending and Transgendering: Male-to-Female Transsexuals, Dichotomy and Diversity', in Gilbert Herdt (ed.), *Third Sex Third Gender, beyond Sexual Dimorphism in Culture and History*, New York, Zone Books, 1996, p. 447.
56. The following sections are readapted from Gross, *Psychology*, pp. 562-75.
57. Electra is another mythological figure in ancient Greece which inspired various works, the most famous of which are probably the tragedies *Electra* by Sophocles and Euripides. Here Electra plans the murder of her mother's lover, who killed her father. Sometimes the term "Oedipus complex" is also used for girls.
58. See also Lesley F. Roberts, Michelle A. Brett, Thomas W. Johnson, and Richard J. Wassersug, 'A Passion for Castration: Characterizing Men Who Are Fascinated with Castration, but Have Not Been Castrated', *Journal of Sexual Medicine*, 5, 7, 2008, pp. 1669–80.
59. S. Golombok, R. Cook, A. Bish, and C. Murray, 'Families Created by the New Reproductive Technologies: Quality of Parenting and Social and Emotional Development of the Children', *Child Development*, 66, 1995, pp. 285–89; S. Golombok, F. MacCallum, and E. Goodman, 'The "Test-Tube" Generation: Parent–Child Relationships and the Psychological Well-Being of *in vitro* Fertilization Children at Adolescence', *Child Development*, 72, 2001, pp. 599–608; S. Golombok, C. Murray, P. Brinsden, and H. Addalla,

'Social versus Biological Parenting: Family Functioning and Socioemotional Development of Children Conceived by Egg or Sperm Donation', *Journal of Child Psychology and Psychiatry*, 40, 1999, pp. 519–27; S. Golombok, A. Spencer, and M. Rutter, 'Children in Lesbian and Single-Parent Households: Psychosexual and Psychiatric Appraisal', *Journal of Child Psychology and Psychiatry*, 24, 1983, pp. 551–72; S. Golombok, F. Tasker, and C. Murray, 'Children Raised in Fatherless Families from Infancy: Family Relationships and the Socioemotional Development of Children of Lesbian and Single Heterosexual Mothers', *Journal of Child Psychology and Psychiatry*, 38, 1997, pp. 783–91. See also Susan Golombok and Robyn Fivush, *Gender Development*, Cambridge, Cambridge University Press, 1994.

60. An account of gender dysphoria from a psychoanalytic approach can be found in Barbara Gaffney and Paulina Reyes, 'Gender Identity Dysphoria', in Monica Lanyado and Ann Horne (eds.), *The Handbook of Child and Adolescent Psychotherapy: Psychoanalytic Approaches*, 2nd ed., New York, Routledge/Taylor and Francis Group, 2009, pp. 436–50.

61. Calvin H. Haber, 'The Psychoanalytic Treatment of a Preschool Boy with a Gender Identity Disorder', *Journal of the American Psychoanalytic Association*, 39, 1, 1991, pp. 107–29, p. 107 (emphases are mine).

62. Lawrence Kohlberg, 'Cognitive-Developmental Analysis of Children's Sex-Role Concepts and Attitudes', in E. E. Maccoby (ed.), *The Development of Sex Differences*, Stanford, CA, Stanford University Press, 1966, pp.82-173; Lawrence Kohlberg, 'Stage and Sequence: The Cognitive-Developmental Approach to Socialization', in D. A. Goslin (ed.), *Handbook of Socialization: Theory in Research*, Boston, Houghton-Mifflin, 1969; see also Lawrence Kohlberg, *The Philosophy of Moral Development: Essays on Moral Development*, vol. 1, San Francisco, Harper and Row, 1981; Lawrence Kohlberg, 'Moral Development and Behavior', in Thomas Likona (ed.), *Moral Stages and Moralization*, Holt, Rinehart and Winston, CBS College Publishing, 1976.I think the publication place is Holt

63. R. G. Slaby and K. S. Frey, 'Development of Gender Constancy and Selective Attention to Same-Sex Models', *Child Development*, 46, 1975, pp. 839–56.

64. C. L. Martin and C. F. Halverson, 'A Schematic Processing Model of Sex Typing and Stereotyping in Children', *Child Development*, 52, 1981, pp. 1119–34. S.L; Bem, 'Gender schema theory: a cognitive account of sex typing', *Psychological Review*, 88, 1981, pp. 354–64.

65. C. L. Martin and C. F. Halverson, 'The Effects of Sex-Stereotyping Schemas on Young Children's Memory', *Child Development*, 54, 1983. pp. 563–74; C. L. Martin and C. F. Halverson, 'Gender Constancy: A Methodological and Theoretical Analysis', *Sex Roles*, 9, 1983, pp. 775–90; see also R. A. Fabes and C. L. Martin, *Exploring Child Development*, 2nd ed., Boston, Allyn and Bacon, 2003. See also C. L. Martin, D. N. Ruble, and J. Szkrybalo, 'Cognitive Theories of Early Gender Development', *Psychological Bulletin*, 128, 2002, pp. 903–33.

66. An interesting comparative study of gender dysphoria can be found in N. H. Bartlett and P. L. Vasey, 'A Retrospective Study of Childhood Gender-Atypical Behavior in Samoan fa'afafine', *Archives of Sexual Behavior*, 35, 6, 2006, pp. 659–66.

67. Herdt makes an interesting comparative analysis of the Hijra and modern transsexuals. See Gilbert Herdt, 'Introduction: Third Sexes and Third Genders', in Gilbert Herdt (ed.), *Third Sex Third Gender, beyond Sexual Dimorphism in Culture and History*, New York, Zone Books, 1996, pp. 21–81, p. 70.

68. Lorber, *Paradoxes of Gender*.

69. An interesting account may be found in René Grémaux, 'Woman Becomes Man in the Balkans', in Gilbert Herdt (ed.), *Third Sex Third Gender, beyond*

Sexual Dimorphism in Culture and History, New York, Zone Books, 1996, pp. 241–81. Another detailed account may be found in Serena Nanda, 'Hijras: An Alternative Sex and Gender Role in India', in Gilbert Herdt (ed.), *Third Sex Third Gender, beyond Sexual Dimorphism in Culture and History*, New York, Zone Books, 1996, pp. 373–419.

70. Feinberg, *Trans Gender Warriors*, p. 22.
71. Ibid., p. 23.
72. Ibid., in particular chap. 3.
73. Ibid., p. 31.
74. Gross, *Psychology*, p. 573.

NOTES TO CHAPTER 4

1. Parliamentary Assembly of the Council of Europe in Strasburg in January 2010. Online at http://assembly.coe.int/Main.asp?link=/Documents/WorkingDocs/Doc09/EDOC12087.htm. Last accessed 20 June 2011. See also a later report by the Council of Europe, *Combating Discrimination on Grounds of Sexual Orientation or Gender Identity—Council of Europe Standards*, 2011.
2. Online at http://www2.ohchr.org/english/bodies/hrcouncil/17session/resolutions.htm. Last accessed 2 September 2011. See also the UK Government Equalities Office, Transgender e-bulletin no.3 August/September 2011. Online at http://www.homeoffice.gov.uk/publications/equalities/lgbt-equality-publications/e-bulletin/e-bulletin-3?view=Binary. Last accessed 2 September 2011.
3. Baudewijntje P. C. Kreukels and Peggy T. Cohen-Kettenis, 'Puberty Suppression in Gender Identity Disorder: The Amsterdam Experience', *Nature Reviews, Endocrinology*, 7, August 2011, p. 466.
4. J. Morris, *Conundrum*, London, Faber and Faber, 1974, pp. 1–2.
5. D. Di Ceglie, 'Gender Identity Disorder in Young People', *Advances in Psychiatric Treatment*, 6, 2000, p. 460.
6. D. Kotula, 'Jerry', in D. Kotula, and W. E. Parker (eds.), *The Phallus Palace*, Los Angeles, Alyson Publications, 2002, pp. 92–94.
7. P. J. Manners, 'Gender Identity Disorder in Adolescence: A Review of the Literature', *Child and Adolescent Mental Health*, 14, 2, 2009, pp. 62–68.
8. Catherine Bruton, 'Should I Help My 12–Year-Old Get a Sex Change?', *Times*, 21 July 2008. Online at http://www.timesonline.co.uk/tol/life_and_style/health/child_health/article4359432.ece. Last accessed 19 September 2011.
9. The quote is taken from Katherine Cummings, *Katherine's Diary: The Story of a Transsexual*, Melbourne, Heinemann, 1992, p. 209.
10. Frank Lewins, *Transsexualism in Society. A Sociology of Male-to-Female Transsexuals*, Melbourne, MacMillan, 1995, p. 14.
11. American Psychiatric Association (APA), *DSM-IV-TR Diagnostic and Statistical Manual of Mental Disorders. Text Revision*, 4th ed., Washington DC, American Psychiatric Association, 2000.
12. World Health Organization (WHO), *ICD-10 International Statistical Classification of Diseases*, Geneva, World Health Organization, 1992.
13. It should be noted that there is another diagnostic tool, called Diagnostic and Statistical Manual for Primary Care (DSM-PC). The DSM-PC describes GID as "the display of a strong and persistent desire to be of the opposite sex" and "persistent discomfort with is or her sex". As cited in Birgit Moller, Herbert Schreier, Alice Li, and Georg Romer, 'Gender Identity Disorder in

Children and Adolescents', *Current Problems in Pediatric and Adolescent Health Care*, 39, 5, 2009, p. 117.

14. APA, *DSM-V Development*. Online at http://www.dsm5.org/Pages/Default. aspx. Last accessed 20 June 2011.

15. Eric Meininger and Gary Remafedi, 'Gay, Lesbian, Bisexual and Transgender Adolescents', in S. Neinstein Lawrence (ed.), *Adolescent Health Care: A Practical Guide*, Minneapolis, Lippincott Williams and Wilkins, 2008, chap. 40.

16. R. L. Spitzer, 'The Diagnostic Status of Homosexuality in DSM-III: A Reformulation of the Issues', *American Journal of Psychiatry*, 138, 1981, pp. 210–15.

17. An interesting study has also shown that colour preference in children with gender dysphoria is non-conforming. See Sandy W. Chiu, Shannon Gervan, Courtney Fairbrother, Laurel L. Johnson, Allison F. H. Owen-Anderson, Susan J. Bradley, and Kenneth J. Zucker, 'Sex-Dimorphic Color Preference in Children with Gender Identity Disorder: A Comparison to Clinical and Community Controls', *Sex Roles*, 55, 5–6, 2006, pp. 385–95.

18. An online version is available at http://apps.who.int/classifications/apps/icd/icd10online/. Last accessed 20 June 2011.

19. M. Besser, S. Carr, P. T. Cohen-Kettenis, P. Connolly, P. De Sutter, M. Diamond, D. Di Ceglie, Y. Higashi, L. Jones, F. P. M. Kruijver, J. Martin, Z-J. Playdon, D. Ralph, T. Reed, R. Reid, W. G. Reiner, D. Swaab, T. Terry, P. Wilson, and K. Wylie, 'Atypical Gender Development—A Review', *International Journal of Transgenderism*, 9, 1, 2006, pp. 29–44. See also K. J. Zucker, 'Gender Identity Disorder in Children and Adolescents', *Annual Review of Clinical Psychology*, 1, 2005, pp. 467–92.

20. World Professional Association for Transgender Health (WPATH), *Standards of Care for the Health of Transsexual, Transgender, and Gender Nonconforming People, Seventh Version*, WPATH, 2011, p. 2. Online at http://www.wpath.org/documents/Standards per cent20of per cent20Care per cent20V7 per cent20-per cent202011 per cent20WPATH.pdf. Last accessed 3 January 2012.

21. Personal communication.

22. Royal College of Psychiatrists, *Gender Identity Disorders in Children and Adolescents. Guidance for Management*, London, Royal College of Psychiatrists, 1998.

23. D. Di Ceglie, 'Gender Identity Disorder', p. 462.

24. B. Wren, 'Early Physical Intervention for Young People with Atypical Gender Identity Development', *Clinical Child Psychology and Psychiatry*, 5, 2000, pp. 220–31.

25. Simona Giordano, 'Gender Atypical Organisation in Children and Adolescents', in M. Boylan (ed.), *International Public Health Policy and Ethics*, Dordrecht, Springer Science + Business Media B. V., 2008; Simona Giordano, 'Gender Atypical Organisation in Children and Adolescents: Ethico-Legal Issues and a Proposal for New Guidelines', *International Journal of Children's Rights*, 15, 3–4, 2007, pp. 365–90.

26. Kreukels and Cohen-Kettenis, 'Puberty Suppression', p. 466.

27. Fernanda Farias de Albuquerque and M. Janelli, *Princesa*, Rome, Sensibili alle Foglie, 1994.

28. B. Fenner and R. Mananzala, 'Letter to the Hormonal Medication for Adolescent Guidelines Drafting Team', presented at the congress Endocrine Treatment of Atypical Gender Identity Development in Adolescents, London, 19–20 May 2005. See also the Sylvia Riviera Law Project at http://srlp.org/. Last accessed 30 June 2011.

29. K. Clements-Nolle, R. Marx, R. Guzman, and Michell Katz, 'HIV Prevalence, Risk Behaviours, Health Care Use and Mental Health Status of Transgender Persons: Implications for Public Health Intervention', *American Journal of Public Health*, 91, 2001, p. 915. Cited in Meininger and Remafedi, 'Gay, Lesbian, Bisexual and Transgender Adolescents', chap. 40.

30. Gender Identity Research and Education Society, *Guidance on Combating Transphobic Bullying in Schools*, Home Office, 2008. Online at http://www.gires.org.uk/assets/Schools/TransphobicBullying.pdf. Last accessed 20 June 2011.

31. N. Adams, T. Cox, and L. Dunstan, 'I Am the Hate that Dare Not Speak Its Name: Dealing with Homophobia in Secondary Schools', *Educational Psychology in Practice*, 20, 3, 2004, pp. 259–69; see also A. Grossman and A. R. D'Augelli, 'Transgender Youth Invisible and Vulnerable', *Journal of Homosexuality*, 51, 1, 2006, pp. 111–28.

32. Di Ceglie, 'Gender Identity Disorder', p. 466.

33. Joe Delaplaine, '39 Precious Lives Honored', *Workers World*, 4 December 2003. Online at http://www.workers.org/ww/2003/trans1204.php. Last accessed 20 June 2011.

34. D. Di Ceglie, 'Management and Therapeutic Aims in Working with Children and Adolescents with Gender Identity Disorders, and Their Families', in D. Di Ceglie and D. Freedman (eds.), *A Stranger in My Own Body—Atypical Gender Identity Development and Mental Health*, London, Karnac Books, 1998, chap. 12, pp. 185–97, p. 185.

35. The explanation of a similar process in a different situation can be found in S. Giordano, 'Persecutors or Victims? The Moral Logic at the Heart of Eating Disorders', *Health Care Analysis*, 11, 3, 2003, pp. 219–28.

36. The term 'significant others' refers to close people, such as family or close friends, who are influential in a person's development and life.

37. Di Ceglie, 'Management and Therapeutic Aims', p. 194; see also D. Di Ceglie, D. Freedman, S. McPherson, and P. Richardson, 'Children and Adolescents Referred to a Specialist Gender Identity Development Service: Clinical Features and Demographic Characteristics', *International Journal of Transgenderism*, 6, 1, 2002. Online at http://www.symposion.com/ijt/ijtvo06no01_01.htm. Last accessed 20 June 2011. With regard to suicidal ideation in cases of insecurity over one's sexual identity, see Y. Zhao, R. Montoro, K. Igartua, and B. D. Thombs, 'Suicidal Ideation and Attempt among Adolescents Reporting "Unsure" Sexual Identity or Heterosexual Identity Plus Same-Sex Attraction or Behavior: Forgotten Groups?', *Journal of the American Academy of Child and Adolescent Psychiatry*, 49, 2, 2010, pp. 104–13.

38. Di Ceglie, 'Gender Identity Disorder', p. 458.

39. S. Ghosh and L. Walker, 'Sexuality: Gender Identity', *E Medicine*, 2006. Online at http://www.emedicine.com/ped/topic2789.htm. Last accessed 20 September 2011.

40. A. L. C. De Vries, T. A. H. Doreleijers, and P. T. Cohen-Kettenis, 'Disorders of Sex Development and Gender Identity Outcome in Adolescence and Adulthood: Understanding Gender Identity Development and Its Clinical Implications', *Pediatric Endocrinology Reviews*, 4, 4, 2007, pp. 343–51.

41. P. Connolly, 'Transgendered Peoples of Samoa, Tonga and India: Diversity of Psychosocial Challenges, Coping, and Styles of Gender Reassignment', presented at the Harry Benjamin International Gender Dysphoria Association Conference, Ghent, Belgium, 2003.

42. Moller, Schreier, Li, and Romer, 'Gender Identity Disorder', pp. 117–43.

43. Di Ceglie, 'Gender Identity Disorder', p. 458.

44. Madeleine S. C. Wallien, Rene Veenstra, Baudewijntje P. C. Kreukels, and Peggy T. Cohen-Kettenis, 'Peer Group Status of Gender Dysphoric Children: A Sociometric Study', *Archives of Sexual Behavior*, 39, 2, 2010, pp. 553–60.
45. Moller, Schreier, Li, and Romer, 'Gender Identity Disorder', p. 118. See also Grossman and D'Augelli, 'Transgender Youth Invisible', pp. 111–28.
46. GIRES, *Transphobic Bullying in Schools*, 2007. Online at www.gires.org. uk/Web_Page_Assets/frontframeset.htm. Last accessed 30 June 2011.
47. Ian Warwick, Elain Chase, and Peter Aggleton, *Homophobia, Sexual Orientation and Schools: A Review and Implications for Action*, Research Report No. 594, University of London, 2004. Online at www.dfes.gov.uk/research/ data/uploadfiles/RR594.pdf. Last accessed 30 June 2011.
48. GLSEN's *National School Climate Survey Sheds New Light on Experiences of Lesbian, Gay, Bisexual and Transgender (LGBT) Students*, 2005. Online at glsen.org/cgi-bin/iowa/all/library/record/1927.html. Last accessed 30 June 2011.
49. Meininger and Remafedi, 'Gay, Lesbian, Bisexual and Transgender Adolescents', chap. 40.
50. Stephen Whittle, Lewis Turner, and Maryam Al-Alami, 'Engendered Penalties: Transgender and Transsexual People's Experiences of Inequality and Discrimination', *Equality Reviews*, 2007. Online at http://www.theequalitiesreview.org.uk/upload/assets/www.theequalitiesreview.org.uk/transgender.pdf. Last accessed 30 June 2011. See also Bernard Reed, Stephenne Rhodes, Pietà Schofield, and Kevan Wylie, *Gender Variance in the UK: Prevalence, Incidence, Growth and Geographic Distribution*, London, GIRES, 2009, p. 19.
51. Meininger and Remafedi, 'Gay, Lesbian, Bisexual and Transgender Adolescents', chap. 40.
52. Personal communication.
53. Online at http://www.libdems.org.uk/campaigns/stop-homophobic-bullying. html http://www.outwest.org.uk/news.php. Last accessed 30 June 2011.
54. R. Hall Horace, 'Teach to Reach: Addressing Lesbian, Gay, Bisexual and Transgender Youth Issues in the Classroom', *New Educator*, 2, 2006, p. 150.
55. Department of Health, *Stand Up for Us: Challenging Homophobia in Schools*, 2007, p. 3. Online at http://www.wiredforhealth.gov.uk/PDF/ stand_up_for_us_04.pdf. Last accessed 30 June 2011.
56. D. Di Ceglie, 'Management and Therapeutic Aims', p. 194; see also Di Ceglie, Freedman, McPherson, and Richardson, 'Children and Adolescents'.
57. Whittle, Turner, and Al-Alami, 'Engendered Penalties'.
58. Di Ceglie, 'Management and Therapeutic Aims', p. 194; see also Di Ceglie, Freedman, McPherson, and Richardson, 'Children and Adolescents'.
59. Clements-Nolle, Marx, Guzman, and Katz, 'HIV Prevalence', p. 915. Cited in Meininger and Remafedi, 'Gay, Lesbian, Bisexual and Transgender Adolescents', chap. 40.
60. Meininger and Remafedi, 'Gay, Lesbian, Bisexual and Transgender Adolescents', chap. 40.
61. Whittle, Turner, and Al-Alami, 'Engendered Penalties'.
62. Reed, Rhodes, Schofield, and Wylie, *Gender Variance in the UK*, p. 4.
63. Di Ceglie, 'Gender Identity Disorder', pp. 458–66; Kenneth J. Zucker and Anne A. Lawrence, 'Epidemiology of Gender Identity Disorder: Recommendations for the Standards of Care of the World Professional Association for Transgender Health', *International Journal of Transgenderism*, 11, 1, 2009, pp. 8–18.

64. Richard Green, 'Gender Identity Disorder in Children and Adolescents', in Michael G. Gelder, Nancy C. Andreasen, Juan J. Lopex-Ibor, and John R. Geddes (eds.), *New Oxford Textbook of Psychiatry*, 2nd ed., Oxford, Oxford University Press, 2009, chap. 9.
65. Moller, Schreier, Li, and Romer, 'Gender Identity Disorder', pp. 117–20.
66. For an account of psychosexual outcome in transsexual women, see S. Weyers, E. Elaut, P. De Sutter, J. Gerris, G. T'sjoen, G. Heylens, G. De Cuypere, and H. Verstraelen, 'Long-Term Assessment of the Physical, Mental, and Sexual Health among Transsexual Women', *Journal of Sexual Medicine*, 6, 3, 2009, pp. 752–60.
67. Moller, Schreier, Li, and Romer, 'Gender Identity Disorder', pp. 117–43.
68. D. Di Ceglie, 'The Organisation of the Gender Identity Development Specialist Service. The Network Model', presented Saturday, 5 March 2005, San Camillo Hospital Rome.
69. Reed, Rhodes, Schofield, and Wylie, *Gender Variance in the UK*, p. 5.
70. Personal communication from specialists working in various clinics.
71. Reed, Rhodes, Schofield, and Wylie, *Gender Variance in the UK*, p. 12.
72. M. S. C. Wallien and P. T. Cohen-Kettenis, 'Psychosexual Outcome of Gender Dysphoric Children', *Journal of American Academy of Child and Adolescent Psychiatry*, 47, 2008, pp. 1413–23.
73. K. J. Zucker and S. J. Bradley, *Gender Identity Disorder and Psychosexual Problems in Children and Adolescents*, New York, Guilford Press, 1995.
74. K. D. Drummond, S. J. Bradley, M. Badali-Peterson, and K. J. Zucker, 'A Follow-Up Study of Girls with Gender Identity Disorder', *Developmental Psychology*, 44, 2008, pp. 34–45.
75. K. J. Zucker, 'On the "Natural History" of Gender Identity Disorder in Children', *Journal of American Academy of Child and Adolescent Psychiatry*, 47, 12, 2008, p. 1362; see also Kenneth J. Zucker and Richard Green, 'Psychosexual Disorders in Children and Adolescents', in Gillian Einstein (ed.), *Sex and the Brain*, Cambridge, MA, MIT Press, 2007, pp. 739–66. This article originally appeared in *Journal of Child Psychology and Psychiatry*, 33, 1, 1992, pp. 107–51.
76. Wallien and Cohen-Kettenis, 'Psychosexual Outcome', p. 1413; another informative and comprehensive study of gender dysphoria can be found in Kenneth J. Zucker and Peggy T. Cohen-Kettenis, 'Gender Identity Disorder in Children and Adolescents', in David L. Rowland and Luca Incrocci (eds.), *Handbook of Sexual and Gender Identity Disorders*, Hoboken, NJ, John Wiley and Sons, 2010, pp. 376–422.
77. Wallien and Cohen-Kettenis, 'Psychosexual Outcome', p. 1414.
78. Ibid.; Zucker, 'On the "Natural History"', p. 1362. It is interesting to note that Wallien and Cohen-Kettenis report that many desisters felt that their cross-gender preferences subsided at entrance in the secondary school. The reasons for this being a 'turning point' are not clear. One consideration may be useful here: I will criticise later in the book the classification of gender dysphoria as a mental illness. However, it is important to note that the use of the DSM-IV criteria may be important to predict the outcome of the children with gender dysphoria and to determine the right time to commence treatment. In this sense, the tools offered by the DSM-IV are valuable and need to be utilised in formats that are different from the psychiatric diagnosis. I will discuss this in Chapter 8. An example of questionnaires for children and adults with gender dysphoria can be found in J. J. Deogracias, L. L. Johnson, H. F. L. Meyer-Bahlburg, S. J. Kessler, J. M. Schober, and K. J. Zucker, 'The Gender Identity/Gender Dysphoria Questionnaire for Adolescents and Adults', *Journal of Sex Research*, 44, 4,

2007, pp. 370–79; see also M. S. C. Wallien, L. C. Quilty, T. D. Steensma, D. Singh, S. L. Lambert, A. Leroux, A. Owen-Anderson, S. J. Kibblewhite, S. J. Bradley, P. T. Cohen-Kettenis, and K. J. Zucker, 'Cross-National Replication of the Gender Identity Interview for Children', *Journal of Personality Assessment*, 91, 6, 2009, pp. 545–52.
79. Wallien and Cohen-Kettenis, 'Psychosexual Outcome', pp. 1413–14.
80. Ibid., p. 1421.
81. Zucker, 'On the "Natural History"', p. 1362.
82. Di Ceglie, Freedman, McPherson, and Richardson, 'Children and Adolescents'.
83. This account is readapted from Moller, Schreier, Li, and Romer, 'Gender Identity Disorder', pp. 117–43.
84. A. B. Wisniewski, K. D. Kirk, and K. C. Copeland, 'Long-Term Psychosexual Development in Genetic Males Affected by Disorders of Sex Development (46,XY DSD) Reared Male or Female', *Current Pediatric Reviews*, 4, 4, 2008, pp. 243–49.
85. M. S. C. Wallien, K. J. Zucker, T. D. Steensma, and P. T. Cohen-Kettenis, '2D:4D Finger-Length Ratios in Children and Adults with Gender Identity Disorder', *Hormones and Behavior*, 54, 3, 2008, pp. 450–54. Here the authors explore the relationship between gender dysphoria and 2D:4D finger ratio. Prenatal testosterone seem to affect the 2D:4D finger ratio in humans, and it also seems that prenatal testosterone may affect gender identity differentiation. The authors conclude that, if this is true, then there would be an association between the 2D:4D ratio and gender identity. They indeed note that women (although not men) with Gender Identity Disorder have a more masculinised finger ratio than the control group.
86. Hideyuki Nawata, Koji Ogomori, Mariko Tanaka, Ryoji Nishimura, Hajime Urashima, Rika Yano, Koichi Takano, and Yasuo Kuwabara, 'Regional Cerebral Blood Flow Changes in Female to Male Gender Identity Disorder', *Psychiatry and Clinical Neurosciences*, 64, 2, 2010, pp. 157–16; see also Frank P. M. Kruijver, Jiang-Ning Zhou, Chris W. Pool, Michel A. Hofman, Louis J. G. Gooren, and Dick F. Swaab, 'Male-to-Female Transsexuals Have Female Neuron Numbers in a Limbic Nucleus', in Gillian Einstein (ed.), *Sex and the Brain*, Cambridge, MA, MIT Press, 2007, pp. 781–90.
87. Eshter Gomez-Gil, Isabel Esteva, Cruz M. Almaraz, Eduardo Pasaro, Santiago Segovia, and António Guillamon, 'Familiality of Gender Identity Disorder in Non-Twin Siblings', *Archives of Sexual Behavior*, 39, 2, 2010, pp. 546–52. See also H. Ujike, K. Otani, M. Nakatsuka, K. Ishii, A. Sasaki, T. Oishi, T. Sato, Y. Okahisa, Y. Matsumoto, Y. Namba, Y. Kimata, and S. Kuroda, 'Association Study of Gender Identity Disorder and Sex Hormone-Related Genes', *Progress in Neuro-Psychopharmacology and Biological Psychiatry*, 33, 7, 2009, pp. 1241–44; C. E. M. Van Beijsterveldt, J. J. Hudziak, and D. I. Boomsma, 'Genetic and Environmental Influences on Cross-Gender Behavior and Relation to Behavior Problems: A Study of Dutch Twins at Ages 7 and 10 Years', *Archives of Sexual Behavior*, 35, 6, 2006, pp. 647–58.
88. J. D. Wilson, 'Hormones and Sexual Behavior', *Endocrinologist*, 13, 2003, p. 208.
89. Moller, Schreier, Li, and Romer, 'Gender Identity Disorder', pp. 117–43.
90. The stria terminalis is a band of fibres that form a part of the hypothalamus.
91. The putamen is a round structure found in the brain.
92. Kreukels and Cohen-Kettenis, 'Puberty Suppression', p. 466.
93. Whittle, Turner, and Al-Alami, 'Engendered Penalties'.

94. Personal communication.

NOTES TO CHAPTER 5

1. "E per tutti il dolore degli altri è dolore a metà", from F. De André and I. Fossati, 'Disamistade', in F. De André and I. Fossati (eds.,), *Anime Salve*, Milan, Ricordi, 1996. My translation.
2. Parts of this chapter rely on previous research. See Simona Giordano, 'Gender Atypical Organisation in Children and Adolescents: Ethico-Legal Issues and a Proposal for New Guidelines', *International Journal of Children's Rights*, 15, 3–4, 2007, pp. 365–90; Simona Giordano, 'Gender Atypical Organisation in Children and Adolescents', in Michael Boylan (ed.), *International Public Health Policy and Ethics*, **Dordrecht**, Springer, 2008, chap. 14, pp. 249–72; Simona Giordano, 'Lives in a Chiaroscuro. Should We Suspend the Puberty of Children with Gender Identity Disorder?', *Journal of Medical Ethics*, 34, 8, 2008, pp. 580–86. I wish to thank Peggy Cohen-Kettenis for his extensive comments on this chapter.
3. Birgit Moller, Herbert Schreier, Alice Li, and Georg Romer, 'Gender Identity Disorder in Children and Adolescents', *Current Problems in Pediatric and Adolescent Health Care*, 39, 5, 2009, pp. 117–43.
4. Ibid.
5. The following account relies on the synthesis offered by ibid.
6. Ibid.
7. Darryl B. Hill, Edgardo Menvielle, Kristin M. Sica, and Alisa Johnson, 'An Affirmative Intervention for Families with Gender Variant Children: Parental Ratings of Child Mental Health and Gender', *Journal of Sex & Marital Therapy*, 36, 1, 2010, pp. 6–23.
8. Baudewijntje P. C. Kreukels and Peggy T. Cohen-Kettenis, 'Puberty Suppression in Gender Identity Disorder: The Amsterdam Experience', *Nature Reviews, Endocrinology*, 7, August 2011, p. 467.
9. M. S. C. Wallien, S. H. M. Van Goozen, and P. T. Cohen-Kettenis, 'Physiological Correlates of Anxiety in Children with Gender Identity Disorder', *European Child and Adolescent Psychiatry*, 16, 5, 2007, pp. 309–15.
10. Moller, Schreier, Li, and Romer, 'Gender Identity Disorder', pp. 117–43.
11. For references see ibid.
12. Reid Vanderburgh, 'Appropriate Therapeutic Care for Families with Pre-Pubescent Transgender/Gender-Dissonant Children', *Child and Adolescent Social Work Journal*, 26, 2, 2009, pp. 135–54.
13. World Professional Association for Transgender Health (WPATH), *Standards of Care for the Health of Transsexual, Transgender, and Gender Nonconforming People*, Seventh Version, WPATH, 2011, pp. 8–9, and p. 29. Online at http://www.wpath.org/documents/Standards per cent20of per cent20Care per cent20V7 per cent20–per cent202011 per cent20WPATH. pdf. Last accessed 3 January 2012.
14. H. F. L. Meyer-Bahlburg, 'Gender Identity Disorder in Young Boys: A Parent- and Peer-Based Treatment Protocol', *Clinical Child Psychology and Psychiatry*, 7, 2002, pp. 360–76.
15. See also A. Dreger, 'Gender Identity Disorder in Childhood: Inconclusive Advice to Parents', *Hastings Center Report*, 39, 1, 2009, pp. 26–29; S. Gilbert, 'Children's Bodies, Parents' Choices', *Hastings Center Report*, 39, 1, 2009, pp. 14–15.
16. See, for example, D. Di Ceglie and E. C. Thummel, 'An Experience of Group Work with Parents of Children and Adolescents with Gender Identity Disorder', *Clinical Child Psychology and Psychiatry*, 11, 3, 2006, pp. 387–96.
17. Moller, Schreier, Li, and Romer, 'Gender Identity Disorder', pp. 117–43.

18. L. Fraser, 'Etherapy: Ethical and Clinical Considerations for Version 7 of the World Professional Association for Transgender Health's Standards of Care', *International Journal of Transgenderism*, 11, 4, 2009, pp. 247–63. Cited in WPATH, *Standards of Care*, p. 31.
19. D. Di Ceglie, 'Management and Therapeutic Aims in Working with Children and Adolescents with Gender Identity Disorders, and Their Families', in D. Di Ceglie and D. Freedman (eds.), *A Stranger in My Own Body—Atypical Gender Identity Development and Mental Health*, London, Karnac Books, 1998, pp. 185–97; D. Di Ceglie, 'Gender Identity Disorder in Young People', *Advances in Psychiatric Treatment*, 6, 2000, pp. 458–66.
20. For a later study and proposal, see D. Di Ceglie, 'Engaging Young People with Atypical Gender Identity Development in Therapeutic Work: A Developmental Approach', *Journal of Child Psychotherapy*, 35, 1, 2009, pp. 3–12.
21. P. T. Cohen-Kettenis, H. A. Delemarre-van de Waal, and L. J. G. Gooren, 'The Treatment of Adolescent Transsexuals: Changing Insights', *Journal of Sexual Medicine*, 5, 8, 2008, pp. 1892–97.
22. Royal College of Psychiatrists, *Gender Identity Disorders in Children and Adolescents, Guidance for Management, Council Report CR63*, January 1998. Online at www.rcpsych.ac.uk/publications/cr/cr63.htm, p. 5. Last accessed 30 June 2011.
23. Kevan Wylie, Robert Fung, Claudia Boshier, and Margaret Rotchell, 'Recommendations of Endocrine Treatment for Patients with Gender Dysphoria', *Sexual and Relationship Therapy*, 24, 2, 2009, pp. 175–87.
24. I owe this original classification to Bernard Reed. In a 2007 paper, Richard Green also advises on taking a staged approach, beginning with the more reversible interventions and life experience before moving to irreversible changes. Richard Green, 'Gender Development and Reassignment', *Psychiatry*, 6, 3, 2007, pp. 121–24.
25. Houk and Lee provided an interesting paper on the treatment of gender dysphoric children and adolescents. See C. P. Houk and P. A. Lee, 'The Diagnosis and Care of Transsexual Children and Adolescents: A Pediatric Endocrinologists' Perspective', *Journal of Pediatric Endocrinology and Metabolism*, 19, 2, 2006, pp. 103–9.
26. I am grateful to Professor Mike Besser for this specification.
27. Readapted from http://en.wikipedia.org/wiki/Tanner_stage. The precise development can be measured by assessing testicular and breast development and levels of sex hormones.
28. This test has been subject to criticism. See, for example, Stephen B. Levine, 'Real-Life Test Experience: Recommendations for Revisions to the Standards of Care of the World Professional Association for Transgender Health', *International Journal of Transgenderism*, 11, 3, 2009, pp. 186–93. The latest WPATH Standards of Care does not refer to Real Life Experience, and recommends that therapeutic options may include "changes in gender expression and role (which may involve living part time or full time in another gender role, consistent with one's gender identity)"; see WPATH, *Standards of Care*, p. 9.
29. BSPED, *Guidelines for the Management of Gender Identity Disorder (GID) in Adolescents and Children. Specific Endocrinological Recommendations*, 2006. Online at http://www.bsped.org.uk/professional/guidelines/docs/BSPEDGIDguidelines.pdf. These guidelines have now been withdrawn. Last accessed 2006. Royal College of Psychiatrists, *Gender Identity Disorders*.
30. Peggy T. Cohen-Kettenis, 'Pubertal Delay as an Aid in Diagnosis and Treatment of a Transsexual Adolescent', *European Child and Adolescent Psychiatry*, 7, 1998, pp. 246–48.

31. Henriette A. Delemarre-van de Waal and Peggy T. Cohen-Kettenis, 'Clinical Management of Gender Identity Disorder in Adolescents: A Protocol on Psychological and Paediatric Endocrinology Aspects', *European Journal of Endocrinology*, 155, issue suppl. 1, 2006, pp. 131–37. Online at http://www.eje-online.org/cgi/content/full/155/suppl_1/S131#F2. Last accessed 30 June 2011.
32. WPATH, *Standards of Care*, p.18
33. Ibid.
34. WPATH, *Standards of Care*, pp. 18–19.
35. Ibid., p. 18.
36. Ibid., p.1.
37. Ibid., p. 4.
38. Information on voice and communication therapy may be found in ibid., pp. 52–54.
39. Endocrine Society. Online at http://www.endo-society.org/about/index.cfm. Last accessed 30 June 2011.
40. Wylie C. Hembree, Peggy Cohen-Kettenis, Henriette A. Delemarre-van de Waal, Louis J. Gooren, Walter J. Meyer III, Norman P. Spack, Vin Tangpricha, and Victor M. Montori, 'Endocrine Treatment of Transsexual Persons: An Endocrine Society Clinical Practice Guideline', *Journal of Clinical Endocrinology & Metabolism*, 94, 9, 2009, pp. 3132–54. Online at http://www.endo-society.org/guidelines/final/upload/Endocrine-Treatment-of-Transsexual-Persons.pdf. Last accessed 30 June 2011.
41. The Amsterdam protocol, instead, recommends that early treatment start *no later than* Tanner Stage 2 or 3. See Kreukels and Cohen-Kettenis, 'Puberty Suppression', p. 468.
42. Royal College of Psychiatrists, *Gender Identity Disorders*.
43. Moller, Schreier, Li, and Romer, 'Gender Identity Disorder', p. 117.
44. Information provided personally by specialists.
45. For a discussion of the UK approach to gender issues also see N. Tugnet, J. C. Goddard, R. M. Vickery, D. Khoosal, and T. R. Terry, 'Current Management of Male-to-Female Gender Identity Disorder in the UK', *Postgraduate Medical Journal*, 83, 984, 2007, pp. 638–42.
46. BSPED, *Guidelines*, p. 2. These guidelines have now been withdrawn.
47. Georgina Selby, *Gender Identity Development Service Conducts New Research*, Wednesday, 6 April 2011. Online at http://www.tavistockandportman.nhs.uk/GIDSresearch. Last accessed 1 July 2011. The report reads: "We are carrying out this study because there is not much evidence on the use of hormone blockers in young people. The aim of the research is to look at the psychological and physical effects of blocking sex hormones in young people aged 12–15 and find out if taking part in the study improves the young people's well being". Whereas continued research is useful and will help to answer the questions that still remain open relating to the unforeseen long term consequences of early suspension of puberty, this report is somewhat misleading, in that it suggests that there is a scarcity of data relating to the risks and benefits of so called 'blockers'. This chapter shows that this body of evidence is already conspicuous.
48. Personal communication.
49. FIERCE is an organisation building the leadership and power of lesbian, gay, bisexual, transgender, and queer youth of colour in New York City. Their website is accessible online at http://www.fiercenyc.org/index.php?s=75. Last accessed 18 November 2011. SRLP is a legal aid organisation based in New York City that serves transgender, intersex, and gender non-conforming people. Their website is accessible online at http://srlp.org/. Last accessed 18 November 2011.

50. B. Fenner and R. Mananzala, 'Letter to the Hormonal Medication for Adolescent Guidelines Drafting Team', presented at the congress Endocrine Treatment of Atypical Gender Identity Development in Adolescents, 19–20 May 2005, London. You can also see A. Godano, M. Maggi, E. Jannini, M. C. Meriggiola, E. Ghigo, O. Todarello, A. Lenzi, and C. Manieri, 'SIAMS-ONIG Consensus on Hormonal Treatment in Gender Identity Disorders', *Journal of Endocrinological Investigation*, 32, 10, 2009, pp. 857–64.
51. Delemarre-van de Waal and Cohen-Kettenis, 'Clinical Management, pp. 131–37.
52. Bojan Pancevski, 'Unhappy as a Boy, Kim Became Youngest Ever Transsexual', *Telegraph*, 28 January 2007. Online at http://www.telegraph.co.uk/news/main.jhtml?xml=/news/2007/01/28/wkim28.xml. Last accessed 1 July 2011.
53. P. T. Cohen-Kettenis and F. Pfäfflin, *Transgenderism and Intersexuality in Childhood and Adolescence. Making Choices*, London, Sage Publications, 2003, p. 171.
54. Kreukels and Cohen-Kettenis, 'Puberty Suppression', p. 467.
55. Ibid., p. 468.
56. Delemarre-van de Waal and Cohen-Kettenis, 'Clinical Management', pp. 131–37.
57. I owe this clarification to Terry Reed. See also Cohen-Kettenis and Pfäfflin, *Transgenderism and Intersexuality*, p. 171.
58. Ibid.
59. Kreukels and Cohen-Kettenis, 'Puberty Suppression', p. 467.
60. I. R. Haraldsen, E. Haug, J. Falch, T. Egeland, and S. Opjordsmoen, 'Cross-Sex Pattern of Bone Mineral Density in Early Onset Gender Identity Disorder', *Hormones and Behavior*, 52, 3, 2007, pp. 334–43.
61. Delemarre-van de Waal and Cohen-Kettenis, 'Clinical Management', pp. 131–37; Kreukels and Cohen-Kettenis, 'Puberty Suppression', p. 470.
62. Information kindly offered by Cohen-Kettenis, personal communication. A history of the approach used in Amsterdam can be found in Kreukels and Cohen-Kettenis, 'Puberty Suppression', pp. 466–72.
63. Personal communication with the specialists. For more, see Delemarre-van de Waal and Cohen-Kettenis, 'Clinical Management', pp. 131–37.
64. Delemarre-van de Waal and Cohen-Kettenis. 'Clinical Management', pp. 131–37.
65. P. T. Cohen-Kettenis and H. Delemarre-van de Waal, 'Clinical Management of Adolescents with Gender Dysphoria', presented at the congress Endocrine Treatment of Atypical Gender Identity Development in Adolescents, 19–20 May 2005, London.
66. P. De Sutter, 'Adolescents and GID. Fertility Issues', presented at the congress Endocrine Treatment of Atypical Gender Identity Development in Adolescents, 19–20 May 2005, London; P. De Sutter, 'Reproductive Options for Transpeople: Recommendations for Revision of the WPATH's Standards of Care', *International Journal of Transgenderism*, 11, 3, 2009, pp. 183–85.
67. De Sutter, 'Adolescents and GID'.
68. Other detailed information relating to reproductive health may be found in WPATH, *Standards of Care*, pp. 50–52.
69. Houk and Lee, 'Diagnosis and Care', pp. 103–9.
70. N. Spack, 'An Endocrine Perspective on the Care of Transgender Adolescents', presented at the 55th annual meeting of the American Academy of Child and Adolescent Psychiatry, 28 October–2 November 2008. Cited in Moller, Schreier, Li and Romer, 'Gender Identity Disorder', pp. 117–43. See also C. Imbimbo, P. Verze, A. Palmieri, N. Longo, F. Fusco, D. Arcaniolo, and V. Mirone, 'A Report

from a Single Institute's 14-Year Experience in Treatment of Male-to-Female Transsexuals', *Journal of Sexual Medicine*, 6, 10, 2009, pp. 2736–45. These authors report that half of the applicants had serious suicidal ideation and that 4 per cent actually attempted suicide. Psychosexual and social outcome was positive after treatment, with 75 per cent of people having better lives after surgery and virtually all being satisfied with their new status and expressing no regret. See also M. H. Murad, M. B. Elamin, M. Z. Garcia, R. J. Mullan, A. Murad, P. J. Erwin, and V. M. Montori, 'Hormonal Therapy and Sex Reassignment: A Systematic Review and Meta-Analysis of Quality of Life and Psychosocial Outcomes', *Clinical Endocrinology*, 72, 2, 2010, pp. 214–31.
71. WPATH, *Standards of Care*, pp. 36–38.
72. An overview of various types of hormones that can be provided may be found in ibid., pp. 48–50.
73. Personal communication.
74. Personal communication.
75. WPATH, *Standards of Care*, p. 47.
76. WPATH, *Standards of Care*, p. 40.
77. Editorial on 'Transsexualism', *Lancet*, 338, 1991, p. 604. Cited in Janice G. Raymond, *The Transsexual Empire. The Making of the She-Male*, London, Teachers College Press, 1994, p. xiii.
78. A clear and comprehensive table of risks associated with hormone therapy is available at WPATH, *Standards of Care*, p. 40.
79. Ibid., p. 20.
80. Vladimir Luxuria, *Le favole non dette*, Milan, Bombiani, 2009, p. 201. My translation.
81. Cohen-Kettenis and Delemarre-van de Waal, 'Clinical Management'. See also Imbimbo, Verze, Palmieri, Longo, Fusco, Arcaniolo, and Mirone, 'Report', pp. 2736–45. This study also reports virtually no regret from persons who underwent cross sex surgery; see also G. De Cuypere, E. Elaut, G. Heylens, G. Van Maele, G. Selvaggi, G. T'Sjoen, R. Rubens, P. Hoebeke, and S. Monstrey, 'Long-Term Follow-Up: Psychosocial Outcome of Belgian Transsexuals after Sex Reassignment Surgery', *Sexologies*, 15, 2, 2006, pp. 126–33.
82. See also H. Kuroda, K. Ohnisi, G. Sakamoto, and S. Itoyama, 'Clinicopathological Study of Breast Tissue in Female-to-Male Transsexuals', *Surgery Today*, 38, 12, 2008, pp. 1067–71; see also A. Adelowo, E. E. Weber-LeBrun, and S. B. Young, 'Neovaginectomy Following Vaginoplasty in a Male-to-Female Transgender Patient: A Case Report and Review of Literature', *Journal of Pelvic Medicine and Surgery*, 15, 3, 2009, pp. 101–4; T. Baba, T. Endo, H. Honnma, Y. Kitajima, T. Hayashi, H. Ikeda, N. Masumori, H. Kamiya, O. Moriwaka, and T. Saito, 'Association between Polycystic Ovary Syndrome and Female-to-Male Transsexuality', *Human Reproduction*, 22, 4, 2007, pp. 1011–16.
83. Abnormal narrowing of the passage.
84. WPATH, *Standards of Care*, p. 63.
85. Ibid., p. 64.
86. With regard to the effects of sex reassignment surgery on reproduction, see De Sutter, 'Reproductive Options', pp. 183–85.
87. Cohen-Kettenis and Pfäfflin, *Transgenderism and Intersexuality*. For a further discussion, see S. E. Olsson and A. Moller, 'Regret after Sex Reassignment Surgery in a Male-to-Female Transsexual: A Long-Term Follow-Up', *Archives of Sexual Behavior*, 35, 4, 2006, pp. 501–6.
88. Metaidoioplasty is an alternative to phalloplasty, in which the tissue of the clitoris, enlarged due to the effects of testosterone treatment, is used to create

a phallus. The dimensions of the phallus are reduced as compared to those generally obtained through phalloplasty, but the surgical technique is simpler, shorter, and less expensive; it does not require the insertion of an erectile prosthesis and is more likely to preserve sensation and capacity for orgasm, which, in contrast, may be lost with phalloplasty.

89. I owe this observation to Peggy Cohen-Kettenis.
90. WPATH, *Standards of Care*, p. 21. See also Royal College of Psychiatrists, *Gender Identity Disorders*, p. 6.
91. Daniel Schweimler, 'Argentine Boy Sex Change Approved', *BBC News*, 26 September 2007. Online at http://news.bbc.co.uk/1/hi/world/americas/7013579. stm. Last accessed 1 July 2011.

NOTES TO CHAPTER 6

1. Jacques Brel, *L'anarchia*, translated in Italian by Giuseppe Gennari di Léo Ferré. My translation from the Italian. Online at http://digilander.libero.it/AcomeChiSaiTu/. Last accessed 20 September 2011.
2. Bojan Pancevski, 'Unhappy as a Boy, Kim Became Youngest Ever Transsexual', *Telegraph*, 28 January 2007. Online at http://www.telegraph.co.uk/news/main. jhtml?xml=/news/2007/01/28/wkim28.xml. Last accessed 1 July 2011.
3. Georgina Selby, 'Gender Identity Development Service Conducts New Research'. Online at http://www.tavistockandportman.nhs.uk/GIDSresearch. Last accessed 20 September 2011.
4. An early account may be found in John Harris, 'Biotechnology, Friend or Foe? Ethics and Control', in Anthony Dyson and John Harris (eds.), *Ethics and Biotechnology*, London, Routledge, 1994, chap. 12, pp. 216–29.
5. David Hume, *On Suicide*, 1783. Online at http://www.anselm.edu/homepage/dbanach/suicide.htm. Last accessed June 2010.
6. Maura A. Ryan, 'The New Reproductive Technologies: Defying God's Dominion', *Journal of Medicine and Philosophy*, 20, 4, 1995, pp. 419–38; John Harris and Simona Giordano, 'On Cloning', *The New Routledge Encyclopaedia of Philosophy*, London and New York Edward Craig Edition, 2003.
7. The Johns Hopkins Medical Institutions News, press release, 13 August 1979, p. 2, as quoted in Janice G. Raymond, *The Transsexual Empire. The Making of the She-Male*, London, Teachers College Press, 1994, p. xi.
8. Ibid., p. 9.
9. Ibid., p. 17.
10. Ibid., p. 97.
11. Ibid., chap. 5.
12. Ibid., p. 144.
13. Interview with Fabrizio De André, by Luciano Lanza, 1993. Online at http://solleviamoci.wordpress.com/2009/01/11/speciale-de-andre-con-lintervista-gli-anarchici-i-poeti-gli-altri/. Last accessed 4 August 2011.
14. Raymond, *Transsexual Empire*, p. 16.
15. Ibid., p. 79.
16. Loren Cameron, *Body Alchemy. Transsexual Portraits*, San Francisco, Cleis Press, 1996, p. 81.
17. Raymond, *Transsexual Empire*, p. 79.
18. B. Fenner and R. Mananzala, 'Letter to the Hormonal Medication for Adolescent Guidelines Drafting Team', presented at the congress Endocrine Treatment of Atypical Gender Identity Development in Adolescents, 19–20 May 2005, London.

19. Raymond, *Transsexual Empire*, p. 79.
20. For further references, see Simona Giordano, 'Sex and Gender: Issues of Public Health and Justice', in Michael Boylan (ed.), *The Morality and Global Justice*, Colorado, Perseus Academics, 2011, chap. 18.
21. I owe this important observation to Professor Peter Clayton.
22. Stenvert L. S. Drop, Wouter J. De Waal, and Sabine M. P. F. De Muinck Keizer-Schrama, 'Sex Steroid Treatment of Constitutionally Tall Stature', *Endocrine Review*, 19, 5, 1998, pp. 540–56.
23. Human Fertilisation and Embryology Act 1990, para. 25. Online at http://www.opsi.gov.uk/Acts/acts1990/ukpga_19900037_en_2#pb7–l1g23 Last accessed 14 May 2012
24. Raymond, *Transsexual Empire*, p. 142.
25. I owe this point to Dino Topi.
26. See, for example, Gilber Herdt (ed.), *Third Sex Third Gender. Beyond Sexual Dimorphism in Culture and History*, New York, Zone Books, 1996.
27. Cameron, *Body Alchemy*, p. 94.
28. World Professional Association for Transgender Health (WPATH), *Standards of Care for the Health of Transsexual, Transgender, and Gender Nonconforming People*, Seventh Version, WPATH, 2011, pp. 1-2. Online at http://www.wpath.org/documents/Standards per cent20of per cent20Care per cent20V7 per cent20–per cent202011 per cent20WPATH.pdf. Last accessed 3 January 2012.
29. Ibid., p. 29.
30. Schweimler, 'Argentine Boy Sex Change Approved'.
31. In Chapter 7 we shall discuss how informed consent for research is regulated in some countries. The point raised here is theoretical rather than legal.
32. See, for example, World Medical Association, Declaration of Helsinki (October 2008). Online at http://www.wma.net/e/policy/b3.htm. Last accessed 1 July 2011. A commentary may be found in Simona Giordano, 'The 2008 Declaration of Helsinki: Some Reflections', *Journal of Medical Ethics*, 36, 2010, pp. 598–603.
33. Baudewijntje P. C. Kreukels and Peggy T. Cohen-Kettenis, 'Puberty Suppression in Gender Identity Disorder: The Amsterdam Experience', *Nature Reviews, Endocrinology*, 7, August 2011, p. 469.
34. Ibid., p. 460.
35. The Abortion Act 1967, amended 1990. Online at http://www.legislation.gov.uk/ukpga/1967/87/contents. Last accessed 6 July 2011.
36. *Gillick v. West Norfolk and Wisbech AHA* [1985] 3 All ER 402 at 409 e-h per Lord Fraser (emphases are mine).
37. N. D. Husak, 'Omission, Causation and Liability', *Philosophical Quarterly*, 30, 121, 1980, pp. 318–26.
38. John C. Hall, 'Acts and Omissions', *Philosophical Quarterly*, 39, 157, 1989, pp. 399–408.
39. WPATH, *The Harry Benjamin International Gender Dysphoria Association's Standards of Care for Gender Identity Disorders*, Sixth Version, February 2001, p. 11. Online at http://www.wpath.org/documents2/socv6.pdf. Last accessed 30 June 2011.
40. WPATH, *Standards of Care*, pp. 58–61.
41. Wylie C. Hembree, Peggy Cohen-Kettenis, Henriette A. Delemarre-van de Waal, Louis J. Gooren, Walter J. Meyer III, Norman P. Spack, Vin Tangpricha, and Victor M. Montori, 'Endocrine Treatment of Transsexual Persons: An Endocrine Society Clinical Practice Guideline', *Journal of Clinical Endocrinology & Metabolism*, 94, 9, 2009, pp. 3132–54. Online at http://www.endo-society.org/guidelines/final/upload/Endocrine-Treatment-of-Transsexual-Persons.pdf, p.5. Last accessed 30 June 2011.

42. WHO, *Brasilia Declaration on Ageing*, WHO, 1–3 July 1996. Online at http://www.oneworld.org/helpage/info/brasilia.html). See also United Nations International Year of Older Persons, 1999. Online at http://www.un.org/esa/socdev/iyop/. Last accessed 6 July 2011.

43. Online at http://www.europarl.eu.int/charter/default_en.htm. See also the Convention for the Protection of Human Rights and Fundamental Freedoms as amended by Protocol n. 11, 4 November 1950, art. 14, Prohibition of discrimination. Online at www.echr.coe.int/Convention/webConvenENG.pdf; the Convention for the Rights of the Child (2 September 1990), Preamble. Online at http://www.unhchr.ch/html/menu3/b/k2crc.htm; the European Social Charter (Revised) (3 May 1996), Part IV, Art. E. Online at http://conventions.coe.int/Treaty/EN/Treaties/Html/163.htm. Last accessed 6 July 2011.

44. S. Besson, 'The Principle of Non-Discrimination in the Convention on the Rights of the Child', *International Journal of Children's Rights*, 13, 4, 2005, pp. 433–61.

45. See, for example, Hembree, Cohen-Kettenis, Delemarre-van de Waal, Gooren, Meyer III, Spack, Tangpricha, and Montori, "Endocrine Treatment of Transsexual Persons', pp. 3132–54, in particular 2.5. Other guidelines make similar suggestions.

46. WPATH, *Standards of Care*, pp.59-61. At p.61 an explanation for the rationale of this clause may be found

47. Raymond, *Transsexual Empire*, p. xvii.

NOTES TO CHAPTER 7

1. Jacques Brel, *L'anarchia*, translated by Giuseppe Gennari di Léo Ferré, published online at http://digilander.libero.it/AcomeChiSaiTu/. Last accessed 7 July 2011.

2. As reported at the Claude Cahun Exhibition in Barcelona, December 2011.

3. From now onward I will usually write 'English law' to refer to the law in force in England and Wales.

4. Online at http://www.legislation.gov.uk/ukpga/2004/7/contents. Last accessed 28 August 2011.

5. *Re Alex [2004] FamCA 297*. Reserved files—by court order the file number and names of counsel and solicitors have been suppressed.

6. A commentary can be found in Sheila Jefferys, 'Judicial Child Abuse: The Family Court of Australia, Gender Identity Disorder, and the "Alex" Case', *Women's Studies International Forum*, 29, 1, Jan.–Feb. 2006, pp. 11–12.

7. Margaret Brazier and Emma Cave, *Medicine Patients and the Law*, 5th ed., London, Penguin, 2011, chap. 5.

8. A discussion may be found in Marc Stauch, Kay Wheat, and John Tingle, *Texts, Cases and Materials on Medical Law and Ethics*, 4th ed., London, Routledge, 2012, p. 76.

9. *Bellinger v. Bellinger* [2003] 2 All ER 593.

10. However, by law consent does not necessarily need to be written: it can be given orally or even by action (if I go to my GP complaining of a sore throat and I open my mouth I am implicitly consenting to the GP touching my face to examine me). Brazier and Cave, *Medicine Patients and the Law*, chap. 5.

11. Ibid.

12. Shaun D. Pattinson, *Medical Law and Ethics*, 3rd ed., London, Sweet and Maxwell, 2011, p. 139.

13. A US court decided that a 'prudent patient' test should prevail. See *Canterbruy v. Spence* (1972) 464 f 2D 772 at 780. The Canadian Supreme Court

also rejected the 'professional medical standard' in deciding how much information the doctor should disclose. Similarly the High Court of Australia followed Canada. See *Rogers v. Whittaker* [1993] 4 Med LR 79. For commentary, see Brazier and Cave, *Medicine Patients and the Law*, chap. 5.

14. For a more in-depth discussion, see Pattinson, *Medical Law and Ethics*, pp. 121–30.
15. *Chatterton v. Gerson* [1981] 1 Q. B. 432.
16. With some notable exceptions in cases of 'therapeutic privilege', which does not concern us here. How the civil and criminal law may regard misrepresentation is discussed by Pattinson, *Medical Law and Ethics*, pp. 122–24.
17. *Ms B v. An NHS Trust Hospital* [2002] EWHC Fam 492. Discussed, for example, by Stauch, Wheat, and Tingle, *Texts, Cases and Materials*, p. 104.
18. An account of belief and its effect upon understanding can be found in ibid., pp. 105–6.
19. Colette Chiland, *Exploring Transsexualism*, London, Karnac Books, 2005, pp. 46–47.
20. M. Commander and C. Dean, 'Symptomatic Trans-Sexualism', *British Journal of Psychiatry*, 156, 1990, pp. 894–96.
21. T. D. Steensma, R. Biemond, F. de Boer, and P. T. Cohen-Kettenis, 'Desisting and Persisting Gender Dysphoria after Childhood: A Qualitative Follow-Up Study', *Clinical Child Psychology and Psychiatry*, advance online publication 2011 doi: 10.1177/1359104510378303. Cited in World Professional Association for Transgender Health (WPATH), *Standards of Care for the Health of Transsexual, Transgender, and Gender Nonconforming People*, Seventh Version, WPATH, 2011, p.13. Online at http://www.wpath.org/documents/Standards per cent20of per cent20Care per cent20V7 per cent20– per cent202011 per cent20WPATH.pdf. Last accessed 3 January 2012.
22. Ibid., p. 35 (my emphasis).
23. In Italy, for example, there are two legal 'institutions': inability and interdiction. Inability is partial incapacity. Inability is decided by a judge and has, as a consequence, the declaration of the legal incapacity of the subject to perform acts of extraordinary administration (for example, selling their properties); a curator is appointed to perform these acts on behalf of the incapacitated. A more severe declaration of incapacity is interdiction, again decreed by a judge, which implies the declaration of complete incapacity to both perform acts of ordinary and extraordinary administration. A tutor will be named, which does not support the incapacitated (as in the former case) but is a *substitute* to the incapacitated. See the Civil Code, articles 414–432, amended by the Law n.6, 9 January 2004.
24. *Gillick v. West Norfolk and Wisbech AHA* [1985] 3 All ER 402, HL.
25. Ibid. Cited and discussed by Brazier and Cave, *Medicine Patients and the Law*, chap. 14.19 (Brazier and Cave's 2011 edition is being printed at the time this book is being written. As the final page numbers in the published edition are at this time unknown, I will from here onward refer to the section numbers present in the book, which will assist the reader in identifying the cited passages).
26. [1985] 3 All ER 402 at 409 e-h per Lord Fraser and at 422 g-j per Lord Scarman; See also *R v. D* (1984) 2 A11 ER 449.
27. *Gillick v. West Norfolk and Wisbech AHA* [1986] A.C. 112 at 169. Cited in Pattinson, *Medical Law and Ethics*, p. 179.
28. *Gillick v. West Norfolk and Wisbech AHA* [1986] A.C. 112 at 189 and 174, respectively. Cited in Pattinson, *Medical Law and Ethics*, p. 179.
29. *Re S* (A Minor) (Consent to Medical Treatment) [1994] 2 FLR 1065; *Re E* (A Minor) (Wardship: Medical Treatment) [1993] 1 FLR 386. I owe this point and references to Nishat Hyder.

30. Brazier and Cave, *Medicine Patients and the Law*, chap. 14.20.
31. M. Freeman, 'Rethinking *Gillick*', in M. Freeman (ed.), *Children's Health and Children's Rights*, Leiden, Martinus Nijhoff Publishers, 2006, pp. 201–17.
32. J. Eekelaar, 'The Emergence of Children's Rights', *Oxford Journal of Legal Studies*, 8, 1986, pp. 161–82. A later case which reaffirmed Gillick was *R (on the application of Axon) v. Secretary of State for Health* [2006] EWHC 37 (Admin).
33. See Stauch, Wheat, and Tingle, *Texts, Cases and Materials*, pp. 102–3.
34. *Gillick v. West Norfolk and Wisbech AHA* [1985] 3 All ER 402 at 409 e-h per Lord Fraser and at 422 g-j per Lord Scarman; *F v West Berkshire Health Authority* [1989] 2 All ER 545; see also *State of Tennessee v. Northern* [1978] 563 SW 2 d 197.
35. What is known as "outcome approach", see J. McHale and M. Fox, *Health Care Law*, London, Maxwell, 1997, p. 280; see *St George's Healthcare Trust v. S R v. Collins and others, ex part S* [1998] 3 All ER 673.
36. J. K. Mason and G. T. Laurie, *Mason and McCall Smith's Law and Medical Ethics*, 8th ed., Oxford, Oxford University Press, 2011, see in particular pp. 73–74.
37. For a detailed review of legislation pertaining the minors' right to refuse medical treatment, see Brazier and Cave, *Medicine Patients and the Law*, chap. 14.21.
38. D. DeGrazia, 'Autonomous Agents and Autonomy-Subverting Psychiatric Conditions', *Journal of Medicine and Philosophy*, 19, 3, 1994, pp. 279–98.
39. See, for example, *Re C (adult refusal of treatment)* [1994] 1 All ER 819, and, for comments, see McHale and Fox, *Health Care Law*. See also the MCA 2005. Online at http://www.legislation.gov.uk/ukpga/2005/9/part/1/crossheading/preliminary. Last accessed 21 September 2011.
40. For more detailed discussion of competence and the courts in gender reassignment cases, see M. Jones, 'Adolescent Gender Identity and the Courts', in Michael Freeman (ed.), *Children's Health and Children's Rights*, Leiden, Martinus Nijhoff Publishers, 2006, pp. 121–48. See also S. Whittle and C. Downs, 'Seeking a Gendered Adolescence: Legal and Ethical Problems of Puberty Suppression among Adolescents with Gender Dysphoria', in E. Heinze (ed.), *Children's Rights: Of Innocence and Autonomy*, Aldershot, Dartmouth Press, 2000, chap. 9, pp. 195–208.
41. Baudewijntje P. C. Kreukels and Peggy T. Cohen-Kettenis, 'Puberty Suppression in Gender Identity Disorder: The Amsterdam Experience', *Nature Reviews, Endocrinology*, 7, August 2011, p. 470.
42. Jones, 'Adolescent Gender Identity', pp. 121–48.
43. BMA, *Medical Ethics Today. The BMA's Handbook of Ethics and Law*, 2nd ed., London, BMA, 2004, p. 131. There is a 2009 edition of this handbook, and the updates relating to the 2004 edition are available online at http://www.bma.org.uk/ethics/metupdates.jsp. Last accessed 5 December 2011. A new paper edition is being produced while this book is written. See also General Medical Council, *0–18: Guidance for All Doctors*, 2007. Online at http://www.gmc-uk.org/guidance/ethical_guidance/children_guidance_index.asp. Last accessed 5 December 2011.
44. BMA, *Medical Ethics Today*, p. 131. A version of the Children Act 1989 is available at http://www.opsi.gov.uk/acts/acts1989/ukpga_19890041_en_2#pt1-l1g1. Last accessed 30 June 2011.
45. BMA, *Medical Ethics Today*, p. 133.
46. UNICEF, Convention on the Rights of the Child, Adopted by General Assembly resolution 44/25 of 20 November 1989, Entry into force 2 September 1990, in accordance with article 49. Online at http://www2.ohchr.org/english/law/crc.htm#art2. Last accessed 7 July 2011.

47. A comprehensive commentary can be found in Brazier and Cave, *Medicine Patients and the Law*, chaps. 14.16–14.17.
48. Mason and Laurie, *Mason and McCall Smith's Law and Medical Ethics*, p. 191.
49. If a child's parents refused consent for a treatment her doctor's recommended as being in her best interests, the doctors may apply to the court. Similarly, if both parents and doctors were against a course of treatment that was deemed to be in the best interests of a child, a concerned individual might apply to the court. See *Re D (A Minor) (Wardship: Sterilization) [1976] 2 WLR 279*. I wish to thank Nishat Hyder for this point and reference.
50. WPATH, *Standards of Care*, p.18 (my emphasis).
51. WPATH, *Standards of Care*, p. 21 (my emphasis).
52. Henriette A. Delemarre-van de Waal and Peggy T. Cohen-Kettenis, 'Clinical Management of Gender Identity Disorder in Adolescents: A Protocol on Psychological and Paediatric Endocrinology Aspects', *European Journal of Endocrinology*, 155, issue suppl. 1, 2006, pp. 131–37. Online at http://www.eje-online.org/cgi/content/full/155/suppl_1/S131#F2. Last accessed 30 June 2011. The citation can be found online at p. 6.
53. WPATH, *Standards of Care*, p. 31.
54. Ibid., p. 2.
55. As cited in Mason and Laurie, *Mason and McCall Smith's Law and Medical Ethics*, p. 649.
56. By 'applicant' I mean the person who applies to treatment.
57. Georgina Selby, 'Gender Identity Development Service Conducts New Research'. Online at http://www.tavistockandportman.nhs.uk/GIDSresearch. Last accessed 5 December 2011.
58. Royal College of Paediatrics and Child Health 2000, 180. Cited in Pattinson, *Medical Law and Ethics*, p. 414.
59. Ibid.
60. See also Mason and Laurie, *Mason and McCall Smith's Law and Medical Ethics*, p. 648.
61. EC 2005/28. Cited in Brazier and Cave, *Medicine Patients and the Law*, chap. 15.1.
62. Pattinson, *Medical Law and Ethics*, p. 378.
63. Stauch, Wheat, and Tingle, *Texts, Cases and Materials*, p. 488.
64. Pattinson, *Medical Law and Ethics*, p. 400.
65. Stauch, Wheat, and Tingle, *Texts, Cases and Materials*, p. 489.
66. Pattinson, *Medical Law and Ethics*, p. 417.
67. J Mason and Laurie, *Mason and McCall Smith's Law and Medical Ethics*, p. 648.
68. Pattinson, *Medical Law and Ethics*, p. 417.
69. From Stauch, Wheat, and Tingle, *Texts, Cases and Materials*, pp. 489–91.
70. *Burke v. GMC* [2005] EWCA Civ 1003.
71. *Ann Marie Rogers v. Swindon Primary Care Trust & Secretary of State for Health* [2006] EWCA Civ 392; *R (Linda Gordon) v. Bromley NHS Primary Care Trust* [2006] E.W.H.C. 2462 (Admin).
72. *Simms v. Simms* [2002] EWHC 2734.
73. Ibid. at para 61. Cited and discussed by Pattinson, *Medical Law and Ethics*, p. 415.
74. Stauch, Wheat, and Tingle, *Texts, Cases and Materials*, p. 462.
75. *Simms v. Simms* [2002] EWHC 2734.
76. Pattinson, *Medical Law and Ethics*, p. 415 (my emphasis).
77. Ibid., p. 381.
78. Ibid., p. 380.

79. Ibid., p. 381.
80. A. Plomer, *The Law and Ethics of Medical Research: International Bioethics and Human Rights*, London, Cavendish Publishing, 2005. As cited in Stauch, Wheat, and Tingle, *Texts, Cases and Materials*, p. 462–63.
81. Online at http://www.legislation.gov.uk/ukpga/1989/41/section/1. Last accessed 15 November 2011.
82. BMA, *Medical Ethics Today*, p. 133.
83. *Bolam v. Friern Hospital Management Committee* [1957] 2 All ER 118, [1957] 1 WLR 634.
84. *Bolitho v. City and Hackney HA* [1998] AC 232 at 242, HL.
85. Ibid. at 243, HL.
86. *A v. A Health Authority* [2002] 1 FCR 481, [2002] Fam 213 at para 43; see also *Re A (medical treatment: male sterilisation)* [2000] 1 FCR 193; *A Hospital NHS Trust v. S and others* [2003] Lloyd's Rep Med 137, (2003) 71 BMLR 188 at para 47.
87. Mason and Laurie, *Mason and McCall Smith's Law and Medical Ethics*, p. 82.
88. *Re A (medical treatment: male sterilisation)* [2000] 1 FCR 193; *A Hospital NHS Trust v. S and others* [2003] Lloyd's Rep Med 137, (2003) 71 BMLR 188 at para 47.
89. As cited in Mason and Laurie, *Mason and McCall Smith's Law and Medical Ethics*, p. 82.
90. Online at http://www.legislation.gov.uk/ukpga/2005/9/contents. Last accessed 20 October 2011.
91. As cited in Mason and Laurie, *Mason and McCall Smith's Law and Medical Ethics*, p. 82.
92. General Medical Council, *0–18: Guidance for All Doctors*, 2007. The page on best interests in online at http://www.gmc-uk.org/guidance/ethical_guidance/children_guidance_12_13_assessing_best_interest.asp. Last accessed 5 December 2011.
93. WPATH, *Standards of Care*, p. 2.
94. *Re J (A Minor) (Child in Care: Medical Treatment)* [1992] 2 All ER 614.
95. Mark Lunney and Ken Oliphant, *Tort Law, Text and Material*, Oxford, Oxford University Press, 2008, in particular pp. 111–43.
96. *Burke v. GMC* [2005] EWCA Civ 1003.
97. *Re J (A Minor) (Child in Care: Medical Treatment)* [1992] 2 All ER 614. "The fundamental issue in the appeal is whether the court in the exercise of its inherent power to protect the interests of minors should ever require a medical practitioner or health authority acting by a medical practitioner to adopt a course of treatment which in the bona fide clinical judgment of the practitioner concerned is contra-indicated as not being in the best interests of the patient. I have to say that I cannot at present conceive of any circumstances in which this would be other than an abuse of power as directly or indirectly requiring the practitioner to act contrary to the fundamental duty which he owes to his patient. This, subject to obtaining any necessary consent, is to treat the patient in accordance with his own best clinical judgment" (Lord Donaldson MR).
98. Stauch, Wheat, and Tingle, *Texts, Cases and Materials*, p. 249. They also cite the Australian case of *Lowns v. Woods* [1996] Aust Torts Rep 81–136, in which a doctor, who was in his surgery at the time, was held liable in tort for failing to answer a summons for help from a stranger.
99. See, for example, *Phillips v. William Whiteley Ltd* [1938] 1 All ER 566.
100. *Bolam v. Friern Hospital Management Committee* [1957] 1WLR 582.
101. Ibid., 587–88. A commentary can be found in Brazier and Cave, *Medicine Patients and the Law*, chap. 7.
102. *Bolitho v. Hackney Health Authority* [1997] 3 WLR 1151.

103. Brazier and Cave, *Medicine Patients and the Law*, chap. 7.
104. Stauch, Wheat, and Tingle, *Texts, Cases and Materials*, p. 128.
105. *Barnett v. Chelsea & Kensington Hospital Management Committee* [1968] 1 All ER 1068.
106. Readapted from Tony Hope, Julian Savulescu, and Judith Hendrick, *Medical Ethics and Law. The Core Curriculum*, 2nd ed., London, Churchill Livingstone, 2008, p. 53.
107. Stauch, Wheat, and Tingle, *Texts, Cases and Materials*, p. 273.
108. Ibid., p. 276. It must be noted that the courts have adopted an alternative reasoning on causation in two other cases: *McGhee v. National Coal Board*, [1972] 3 All E.R. 1008, 1 W.L.R. 1, and *Fairchild v. Glenhaven Funeral Services Ltd* [2002] UKHL 22.
109. Lunney and Oliphant, *Tort Law, Text and Material*, pp. 111–43.
110. *Judicial Review: A Short Guide to Claims in the Administrative Court*, Research Paper 28, September 2006. Online at http://www.parliament.uk/documents/commons/lib/research/rp2006/rp06-044.pdf. Last accessed 21 October 2011.
111. Personal communication.
112. WPATH, *Standards of Care*, p. 13, p. 22, p. 41, p. 52, p. 62, respectively, for the various stages of therapy.
113. Ibid.
114. Wylie C. Hembree, Peggy Cohen-Kettenis, Henriette A. Delemarre-van de Waal, Louis J. Gooren, Walter J. Meyer III, Norman P. Spack, Vin Tangpricha, and Victor M. Montori, 'Endocrine Treatment of Transsexual Persons: An Endocrine Society Clinical Practice Guideline', *Journal of Clinical Endocrinology & Metabolism*, 94, 9, 2009, pp. 3132–54. Online at http://www.endo-society.org/guidelines/final/upload/Endocrine-Treatment-of-Transsexual-Persons.pdf, p. 8 online. Last accessed 4 December 2012.
115. WPATH, *Standards of Care*, p. 5.

NOTES TO CHAPTER 8

1. An earlier version of this chapter was published in Simona Giordano, 'Where Christ Did Not Go; Men, Women, and frusculicchi. Epistemological and Ethical Issues Relating to Gender Minorities', *Monash Bioethics Review*, in press.
2. Carlo Levi, *Cristo si è fermato ad Eboli*, Turin, Mondadori, 1985, Introduzione, p.3. English ed. *Christ Stopped at Eboli*, London, Penguin, 2000.
3. Ibid., chap. 1.
4. This is a widely used term in the transgender community. See, for example, http://www.traditionalvalues.org/pdf_files/TVCSpecialRptTransgenders1234.PDF; http://www.malikatv.blogspot.com/2006/04/pakistan-hijras-caught-in-no-mans-land.html. Last accessed 13 May 2011.
5. Online at http://www.un.org/en/documents/udhr/. Last accessed 13 May 2011.
6. Government Equalities Office, 'Transgender E-Bulletin', April/May 2011. Online at http://www.homeoffice.gov.uk/publications/equalities/lgbt-equality-publications/e-bulletin/transgender-ebulletin-1?view=Binary. Last accessed 16 September 2011.
7. World Professional Association for Transgender Health (WPATH), *Standards of Care for the Health of Transsexual, Transgender, and Gender Nonconforming People*, Seventh Version, WPATH, 2011, p. 4. Online at http://

www.wpath.org/documents/Standards of Care V7 – 2011 WPATH.pdf. Last accessed 3 January 2012.

8. Of course, gender transition involves in some ways others and the society at large. Some of the normative implications of this will be discussed in the next chapter.

9. Some interesting debates on this point were made in the debates on gender at the Parliamentary Assembly of the Council of Europe in Strasburg in January 2010. See http://assembly.coe.int/Main.asp?link=/Documents/Working-Docs/Doc09/EDOC12087.htm. Last accessed 13 May 2011.

10. Readapted from American Psychiatric Association, *Summary of Practice-Relevant Changes to the DSM-IV-TR*. Online at http://www.psych.org/MainMenu/Research/DSMIV/DSMIVTR/DSMIVvsDSMIVTR/SummaryofPracticeRelevantChangestotheDSMIVTR.aspx. Last accessed 13 May 2011.

11. H. Stuart, 'Mental Illness and Employment Discrimination', *Current Opinion in Psychiatry*, 19, 5, 2006, pp. 522–26; Ann Bartel and Paul Taubman, 'Some Economic and Demographic Consequences of Mental Illness', *Journal of Labor Economics*, 4, 2, 1986, pp. 243–56.

12. See American Psychiatric Association, *Summary*.

13. See, for example, C. Boorse, 'Concepts of Health', in Donald VanDeveer and Tom Regan (eds.), *Health Care Ethics: An Introduction*, Philadelphia, Temple University Press, 1987, p. 372.

14. These could be relevant, in that if I believe that there is no such a thing as a *mental disorder*, then of course I may contest the inclusion of GID amongst mental disorders on that ground. The epistemological issues raised by psychiatric diagnoses have been widely covered in philosophy of psychiatry or psychiatric ethics, and this chapter does not provide a critique of the notion of mental disorder altogether. For some classic critique, see Tristram H. Engelhardt and Stewart F. Spicker, *Mental Health: Philosophical Perspectives*, Dordrecht, Reidel Publishing, 1976; T. Szasz, *The Myth of Mental Illness*, London, Paladin, 1984; G. Jervis, *Manuale critico di psichiatria*, Milan, Feltrinelli, 1997; R. Boyers, *Laing and Antipsychiatry*, London, Penguin, 1972; David Cooper, *Psychiatry and Antipsychiatry*, London, Paladin, London, 1970; L. A. Sass, *Madness and Modernism*, London, Harvard University Press, 1992.

15. See American Psychiatric Association, *Summary*. See also Jerome C. Wakefield, Kathleen J. Pottick, and Stuart A. Kirk, 'Should the DSM-IV Diagnostic Criteria for Conduct Disorder Consider Social Context?', *American Journal of Psychiatry*, 159, 2002, pp. 380–86.

16. The DSM-IV characterises mental disorders as psychological or behavioral patterns generally associated with distress in the individual or disability, and which are not a part of normal development or culture. The notion of mental disorder includes "clinically significant distress or impairment in social, occupational, or other important areas of functioning". American Psychiatric Association, *Summary*.

17. It is worth noting that the notion of mental disorder/illness is contentious. The DSM-IV Taskforce regards a mental disorder as "clinically significant distress or impairment in social, occupational, or other important areas of functioning". Thus the notion of mental disorder that is currently accepted at least by the American Psychiatric Association includes suffering *or* impairment of social adjustment and functioning. See American Psychiatric Association, *Diagnostic and Statistical Manual of Mental Disorders, DSM-IV*, Washington DC, American Psychiatric Association, 1994, p. 7. For a critical analysis, see R. L. Spitzer and J. C. Wakefield, 'DSM-IV Diagnostic Criterion

for Clinical Significance: Does It Help Solve the False Positives Problem?', *American Journal of Psychiatry*, 156, 1999, pp. 1856–64. There is a fourth 2000 edition of the DSM, known as DSM-IV-TR (Text Revision). Here the clinical significance criterion has been retained. A DSM-IV is due in May 2013. Online at http://www.dsm5.org/Pages/Default.aspx. Last accessed 13 May 2011.

18. Simona Giordano, 'Ethics of Management of Gender Atypical Organisation in Children and Adolescents', in M. Boylan (ed.), *International Public Health Policy and Ethics*, Dordrecht, Springer, 2008, pp. 249–72.

19. T. P. Cohen-Kettenis and F. Pfäfflin, *Transgenderism and Intersexuality in Childhood and Adolescence. Making Choices*, London, Sage Publications, 2003.

20. See http://assembly.coe.int/Main.asp?link=/Documents/WorkingDocs/Doc09/EDOC12087.htm. Last accessed 13 May 2011. Government Equalities Office, 'Transgender E-Bulletin'. For cases of murder of children with GID, see D. Di Ceglie, 'Gender Identity Disorder in Young People', *Advances in Psychiatric Treatment*, 6, 2000, pp. 458–66.

21. A comprehensive account of how social policies and law are often gender/sex biased can be found in C. Kitzinger, 'Sexualities', in Rhoda K. Unger (ed.), *Handbook of the Psychology of Women and Gender*, Hoboken, NJ, Wiley, 2001, chap. 6.

22. In Australia there seems to be the possibility of an "indeterminate gender" passport. Online at http://www.smh.com.au/national/transsexual-wins-apology-over-passport-20091030-hprb.html?autostart=1. See also 'Australian Passports to Have Third Gender Option', *Guardian*, 15 September 2011. Online at http://www.guardian.co.uk/world/2011/sep/15/australian-passports-third-gender-option. Last accessed 20 September 2011.

23. M. S. C. Wallien, K. J. Zucker, T. D. Steensma, and P. T. Cohen-Kettenis, '2D:4D Finger-Length Ratios in Children and Adults with Gender Identity Disorder', *Hormones and Behavior*, 54, 3, 2008, pp. 450–54; Nawata Hideyuki, Ogomori Koji, Tanaka Mariko, Nishimura Ryoji, Urashima Hajime, Yano Rika, Takano Koichi, and Kuwabara Yasuo, 'Regional Cerebral Blood Flow Changes in Female to Male Gender Identity Disorder', *Psychiatry and Clinical Neurosciences*, 64, 2, 2010, pp. 157–61.

24. S. Ghosh and L. Walker, 'Sexuality: Gender Identity', *E Medicine*, 2006. Online at http://www.emedicine.com/ped/topic2789.htm. Last accessed 13 May 2011.

25. A reprint of the DSM-IV criteria can be found online at http://www.behavenet.com/capsules/disorders/genderiddis.htm. Last accessed 13 May 2011.

26. Janice G. Raymond, *The Transsexual Empire. The Making of the She-Male*, New York, Teachers College Press, 1994, p. 6.

27. T. Szasz, *The Myth of Mental Illness*, London, Paladin, 1984.

28. Ibid.

29. Gilbert Ryle, *The Concept of Mind*, London, Penguin, 1978.

30. A. J. Ayer, *Truth and Logic*, London, Penguin, 1990, p. 130. See also P. V. Inwagen, 'Philosophers and the Words "Human Body"', in P. V. Inwagen (ed.), *Time and Cause, Essays Presented to Richard Taylor*, London, Springer, 1980, pp. 283–99. See also Ryle, *Concept of Mind*, p. 15

31. Kiira Triea, *Hasting Center Report, Bioethics Forum*, 2010. Online at http://www.thehastingscenter.org/Bioethicsforum/Post.aspx?id=4426. Last accessed 13 May 2011.

32. See, for example, Boorse, 'Concepts of Health', p. 372.

33. Simona Giordano, 'A Heaven without Giants or Dwarfs', unpublished.

34. Herbert Marcuse, *Repressive Tolerance*, 1965. An online version is available at http://www.marcuse.org/herbert/pubs/60spubs/65repressivetoleranc e.htm. Last accessed 13 May 2011.
35. The speech can be listened in Italian at http://www.youtube.com/ watch?v=2px-6gdD0C8. My translation. Last accessed 15 May 2012
36. P. Connolly, 'Transgendered Peoples of Samoa, Tonga and India: Diversity of Psychosocial Challenges, Coping, and Styles of Gender Reassignment', presented at Harry Benjamin International Gender Dysphoria Association Conference, 2003, Ghent, Belgium.
37. WPATH, *The Harry Benjamin International Gender Dysphoria Association's Standards of Care for Gender Identity Disorders*, Sixth Version, February 2001, p. 6. Online at http://www.wpath.org/documents2/socv6.pdf. Last accessed 30 June 2011.
38. M. S. C. Wallien and P. T. Cohen-Kettenis, 'Psychosexual Outcome of Gender Dysphoric Children', *Journal of the American Academy of Child and Adolescent Psychiatry*, 47, 2008, pp. 1413–23.
39. *AC v. Berkshire West Primary Care Trust* [2010] ACD 75, [2010] EWHC 1162 (Admin), [2010] Med LR 281. See also Adam Wagner, 'Court Rules that NHS Was Right to Reject Transsexual's Breast Enlargement Claim', *Guardian*, 28 May 2010. Online at http://www.guardian.co.uk/law/2010/ may/28/transsexual-nhs-breast-enlargement. Last accessed 13 May 2011.
40. Bernard Reed, Stephenne Rhodes, Pietà Schofield, and Kevan Wylie, *Gender Variance in the UK: Prevalence, Incidence, Growth and Geographic Distribution*, London, Gender Identity Research and Education Society, 2009, p. 20.
41. I owe this observation to Norman Spack.
42. *Syndrome* is a word of Greek origins, which literally means 'running together'.
43. An illness can equally be a part of personal identity, of course. It should also be noted that recognising that a cluster of experiences might be regarded as a syndrome is not incompatible in principle with regarding gender identity development as a normal and nonpathological part of who we are. A syndrome is, strictly speaking, only a cluster of experiences and occurrences that are observed in concomitance.
44. Robin McKie and Gaby Hinsliff, 'This Couple Want a Deaf Child. Should We Try to Stop Them?', *Guardian*, 9 March, 2008. Online at http://www.guardian.co.uk/science/2008/mar/09/genetics.medicalresearc h. Last accessed 31 May 2011.
45. I wish to thank Norman Spack for this information.
46. I use 'cosmetic' in inverted commas for the following reasons: first, it is unclear what it is that makes some interventions 'cosmetic' rather than 'reparative' or 'regenerative', for example. Thus the term appears too imprecise to qualify what it proposes to qualify. Second, the adjective has important normative connotations. It qualifies the intervention as 'nonmedical', as somehow superfluous. This begs the question as to why some types of requests are thought of as based on a 'clinical' necessity whereas others are regarded as based on a somehow more 'arbitrary' preference. Finally, it implies that a claim for 'cosmetic' intervention does not have the same compelling force than a claim based on a 'clinical' need: this assumes somehow what needs demonstrating.
47. I owe this observation to Annabelle Lever.
48. Jervis, *Manuale critico di psichiatria*, chap. 3.
49. GLSEN, *National School Climate Survey Sheds New Light on Experiences of Lesbian, Gay, Bisexual and Transgender (LGBT) Students*, 2005. Online at http://glsen.org/cgi-bin/iowa/all/library/record/1927.html. Last accessed

13 May 2011. See also I. Warwick, E. Chase, and P. Aggleton, *Homophobia, Sexual Orientation and Schools: A Review and Implications for Action*, Research Report No. 594, University of London, 2004. Online at https://www.education.gov.uk/publications/eOrderingDownload/RB594MIG1188.pdf. Last accessed 13 May 2011.
50. *Universal Declaration of Human Rights*. Online at http://www.un.org/en/documents/udhr/. Last accessed 13 May 2011.
51. *Universal Declaration of Human Rights, Preamble*. Online at http://www.un.org/en/documents/udhr/index.shtml. Last accessed 13 May 2011.

NOTES TO CHAPTER 9

1. F. De André and I. Fossati, 'Khorakhané', *Anime Salve*, Milan, Ricordi, 1996. Khorakhané is a group of nomad gypsies of Serbian origin. My translation from the Italian.
2. An earlier version of this chapter was published in Simona Giordano, 'Sliding Doors', *Medicine Healthcare and Philosophy*, forthcoming.
3. Istar Lev Arlene, 'Disordering Gender Identity. Gender Identity Disorder in the DSM-IV-TR', *Journal of Psychology and Human Sexuality*, 17, 3–4, 2006, pp. 35–69; Walter O. Bockting and Randall D. Ehrbar, 'Commentary Gender Variancy, Dissonance or Identity Disorder?', *Journal of Psychology and Human Sexuality*, 17, 3–4, 2006, pp. 125–34.
4. C. A. Ross, 'Ethics of Gender Identity Disorder', *Ethical Human Psychology and Psychiatry*, 11, 3, 2009, pp. 165–70.
5. I use 'medical care', 'intervention', and 'treatment' as synonymous, even if there is no 'illness' to 'cure' in gender dysphoria.
6. I have explained in Chapter 8 why 'cosmetic' is used in inverted commas. See note 45.
7. The source of these pictures is http://www.girlpower.it/look/tendenze/body_modification.php. Last accessed 22 September 2011.
8. E. Kaw, 'Medicalization of Racial Features: Asian American Women and Cosmetic Surgery', *Medical Anthropology Quarterly*, 7, 1, 2003, p. 75.
9. E. Haiken, *Venus Envy. A History of Cosmetic Surgery*, Baltimore, MD, Johns Hopkins University Press, 1997; S. Baumann, 'The Moral Underpinnings of Beauty: A Meaning-Based Explanation for Light and Dark Complexions in Advertising', *Poetics*, 36, 2008, p. 5; C. A. D. Charles, 'Skin-Bleaching, Self-Hate, and Black Identity in Jamaica', *Journal of Black Studies*, 33, 2003, pp. 711–28.
10. M. O. Little, 'Suspect Norms of Appearance and the Ethics of Complicity', in I. de Beaufort, M. Hilhorst, and S. Holm (eds.), *In the Eye of the Beholder: Ethics and Medical Change of Appearance*, Copenhagen, Scandinavian University Press, 1996, pp.151-67; M. O. Little, 'Cosmetic Surgery, Suspect Norms, and the Ethics of Complicity', in E. Parens (ed.), *Enhancing Human Traits: Conceptual Complexities and Ethical Implications*, Washington DC, Georgetown University Press, 1998, pp.162-76.
11. I put *racial* in inverted commas because the qualification of a medical intervention as 'racial' implies a morally negative connotation, and thus the adjective somewhat begs the question as to why these interventions are regarded as 'racial' and therefore morally controversial. In this chapter by 'racial' I refer to those interventions that seek to temper features associated with one's ethnic origins. In this chapter the case of 'racial' surgery is only used to illustrate an instance of an ethically controversial medical procedure.

12. C. Kitzinger, 'Sexualities', in Rhoda K. Unger (ed.), *Handbook of the Psychology of Women and Gender,* Hoboken, NJ, Wiley, 2001.

13. J. Lorber, *L'invenzione dei sessi,* Milan, Il Saggiatore, 1995, p. 40.

14. W. K. Scott, 'Gender: A Useful Category of Historical Analysis', *American Historical Review,* 91, 5, 1986, pp. 1053–75. Online at http://www.cedis. uni-koeln.de/content/e310/e625/Text1frWorkshopzurHermeneutischenDialoganalyse_gender_ger.pdf. Last accessed 11 June 2011.

15. BMA, *Eating Disorders, Body Image & the Media,* London, BMA, 2000, p. 43.

16. CCN, 13 September 2006. Online at http://www.cnn.com/2006/WORLD/europe/09/13/spain.models/index.html. Last accessed 11 June 2010.

17. By *authenticity* here I mean the extent to which these wishes are formed autonomously and are not purely the result of social conditioning. It is not clear whether this could be understood, but this is also why it should not be doctors to judge how to treat on this basis.

18. Stenvert L. S. Drop, Wouter J. De Waal, and Sabine M. P. F. De Muinck Keizer-Schrama, 'Sex Steroid Treatment Of Constitutionally Tall Stature', *Endocrine Review,* 19, 5, 1998, pp. 540–56.

19. Of course, in this case, one should also accept that doctors be in charge of resolving the epistemic problem of determining the degree in which the request is 'socially' determined and the moral problem of deciding when the request is 'too' socially constructed to deserve medical attention.

20. I owe this observation to Charles Erin.

21. United Nations, *Universal Declaration of Human Rights,* 1948. Online at http://www.un.org/en/documents/udhr/. Last accessed 11 June 2011.

22. References available in scenario 1.

23. S. Giordano, 'Gender Atypical Organisation in children and Adolescents: Ethico-Legal Issues and a Proposal for New Guidelines', *International Journal of Children's Rights,* 15, 3–4, 2007, pp. 365–90.

24. T. Hope, J. Savulescu and J. Hendrick, *Medical Ethics and Law, the Core Curriculum,* London, Churchill Livingstone, 2008, chap. 9.

25. BBC News, *Body Dysmorphic Disorder,* 2000. Online at http://news.bbc. co.uk/2/hi/health/medical_notes/625913.stm. Last accessed 11 June 2011.

26. Drop, De Waal, De Muinck Keizer-Schrama, 'Sex Steroid Treatment ', pp. 540–56.

27. I owe this observation to Peter Clayton.

28. S. Giordano 'A heaven without Giants or Dwarfs: Equality, Gender and Disabilities', unpublished.

29. R. McKie and G. Hinsliff, 'This Couple Want a Deaf Child. Should We Try to Stop Them?', *Guardian,* 9 March 2008. Online at http://www.guardian. co.uk/science/2008/mar/09/genetics.medicalresearch. Last accessed 11 June 2011.

30. P. J. Manners, 'Gender Identity Disorder in Adolescence: A Review of the Literature', *Child and Adolescent Mental Health,* 14, 2, 2009, pp. 62–68.

31. B. Moller, H. Schreier, A. Li, and G. Romer, 'Gender Identity Disorder in Children and Adolescents', *Current Problems in Pediatric and Adolescent Health Care,* 39, 5, 2009, pp. 117–43.

32. This is an example of how this works: in 2010, in Italy, in a family with a cumulative income of over 40,000 euros per year, a dermatological visit at a specialist clinic costs 24 euros (against anything between 60 and 150 euros in the private sector, and in addition to normal yearly tax based on income). Families with a cumulative salary of less than 40,000 euros will be exempt.

NOTES TO CHAPTER 10

1. As Reported at the Claude Cahun Exhibition in Barcelona, December 2011.
2. Renzo Novatore, *My Iconoclastic Individualism*, 1920. Online at http://theanarchistlibrary.org/HTML/Renzo_Novatore__My_Iconoclastic_Individualism.html. Last accessed 12 January 2012.
3. Jean Jacques Rousseau, *Discours sur l'origine et les fondements de l'inégalité parmi les hommes*, 1755. A translation by G. D. H. Cole of this discourse, also known as *Discourse on Equality*, is online at http://www.munseys.com/diskone/ineq.pdf. Last accessed 17 January 2012.
4. The quote can be found in Richard Wall, 'The Radical Individualism of Paul Goodman'. Online at http://www.lewrockwell.com/orig3/wall10.html. Last accessed 12 January 2012.
5. Issue of *Workers World*, 4 December 2003. Online at http://www.workers.org/ww/2003/trans1204.php. Last accessed 17 January 2012.
6. J. J. C. Smart and B. Williams, *Utilitarianism: For and Against*, Cambridge, Cambridge University Press, 1996, p. 28.

Index